400 METERS

To join the conversation
on how *400 Meters*
can help change the lives
of people experiencing
depression, connect with
Forest on Facebook
@400meters or at
400metersthebook@gmail.com.

400 METERS

A PERSONAL TALE OF OVERCOMING DEPRESSION

FOREST RUNNELS

AUTHOR / PUBLISHER

400 METERS

A PERSONAL TALE OF OVERCOMING DEPRESSION

Written and published by Forest Runnels.
Copyright © 2019 by Forest Runnels.

ISBN: 9781673570571

This book is dedicated to my two wonderful grandmothers who passed away in 2016. May your beautiful souls rest in peace.

Cheryl Mae Osborne
April 9, 1958 – April 8, 2016

Pamela Lee Runnels
May 9, 1953 – November 21, 2016

TABLE OF CONTENTS

Preface 9

Chapter 1: Beginning of the End 11

Chapter 2: Thumbs Up 15

Chapter 3: When it Rains, It Pours 19

Chapter 4 : Pain, Pain Go Away 25

Chapter 5: Breathe 29

Chapter 6: The Moment of Truth 33

Chapter 7: Promises Made 39

Chapter 8: Don't Let Me Miss You 43

Chapter 9: Gasping for Air 47

Chapter 10: Digging Deep 53

Chapter 11: Call to Action 59

Chapter 12: Fatherly Advice 65

Chapter 13: The Road Home 71

Chapter 14: Breathing Fresh Air 77

Chapter 15: Back to the Track 83

Chapter 16: Taking a Chance 89

Chapter 17: A New Beginning 97

Chapter 18: Holy 101

Epilogue 113

Acknowledgements 117

About the Author 121

PREFACE

The following is a true story with the acknowledgment that I am nothing but grateful for the life I have been given. I have two loving parents who have always been very supportive of me. I have a sister, who despite being a goofball, is a good person that has always looked up to me. I have a beautiful wife named Brittany; she's been such a blessing since our first date. And I have two wonderful grandfathers who would do anything for me. I also have the cutest dog in the world. Add to this a college degree and the fact that I landed a good job when I graduated. Sounds like a nice life, right? If you think so, I agree.

However, that doesn't mean life hasn't come without struggles or tough times. There was roughly a four-month period of my life that made me question so many things and wonder what my purpose in the world was. These four months required me to pull something out of myself in order for the blessings I mentioned above to come to fruition.

I give 99% of the credit to overcoming those four months to the people mentioned above, but it literally took me being knocked down over-and-over again to find that missing 1%. This 1% led me to understand that life is *always* worth living, and there are always reasons to keep your head up and not give up.

The following narrative is a portrayal of how I managed to make it through a rough time in my personal life. The names of certain people have been changed for the purpose of anonymity. This story is to help those struggling with depression, illness, grief, or dealing with betrayal in a relationship. I sincerely hope it can help with any and all issues one could be facing, but these are the four topics I mainly touch upon.

CHAPTER 1: BEGINNING OF THE END

It was late February 2016, and I was a sophomore in college. I attended Wright State University in Fairborn, Ohio majoring in Political Science. I know, go ahead and insert the "Arts Degrees are worthless" comments. At the time, I was just getting into my major-specific classes and had completed my Common Core or general education classes the semester before. School was always something I had a knack for. It always came easy to me because I am a person that genuinely loves to learn.

As one would expect from a person that said that school comes easy to them, I was doing just fine in my classes, and I managed to get to Spring Break with straight A's without much trouble. It was quite a good feeling that I didn't have to worry about school during Spring Break. Since I had a week away from school, I had planned a small weekend trip to Tennessee with my girlfriend Sophia.

The trip could only be for the weekend because I was a cashier at a local Marathon gas station, and I was only able to request off for that weekend because we had such a small staff that it was hard to get time off for part-time workers like myself. I didn't mind that I had to return to work, though, because I wanted the money, and I really couldn't afford to have any longer of a trip at the time anyways.

You're probably expecting me to give a description of the trip next, but I'll be honest, it's not worth the time. The only thing worth mentioning from the trip is that Sophia and I spent a considerable amount of time being quiet or bickering. Things of that nature are common when you're with someone for 6 years.

However, something felt different about the bickering this time. It felt like more than that, but when you're young in a relationship, part of you is scared to acknowledge issues like that, so you just kind of ignore it and pretend it is okay. That is precisely what we did.

We arrived back home after a long drive of silence; she gazed at me with a strange look in her eyes I hadn't seen before. She then said to me that she believed that we should take a "break." Even though I had felt something along the lines of this coming, it was still a bit of a shock. Our relationship had been on the rocks for roughly a year primarily because of her always wanting attention from anyone but me and then getting upset at me when I was upset with that idea. That coupled with me seeing text message conversations between her and a couple other guys did not necessarily help me to trust her.

Despite this, it was still a shock regardless of how much I subconsciously suspected it. She told me that she had been feeling this way for roughly a year and just now decided that it might be best if we separate for a while. I admit, I was upset, but at that moment I wasn't particularly scared because we had been on "breaks" before, and they never lasted more than a couple days.

I drove home wondering what I did to cause this. Don't get me wrong, I made my share of mistakes. Everyone makes mistakes in relationships when you're young, but I genuinely felt that she was the one causing the rift between us, and I was trying to look past it. Yet she was the one that wanted some sense of separation? Fine, so be it.

I drove home in silence as I really wasn't in the mood for music or any noise for that matter. It felt as if that could make me exponentially angrier than I already was. To my annoyance, the silence was broken by a phone call from my mother. She seemed really down, so I asked her what was wrong. She told me my Grandma Cheryl (her mother) had become very sick and was taken to the hospital, so I decided to re-route where I was going and head to meet my family at the hospital.

I arrived roughly a half-hour later to see my grandma lying in a hospital bed. She had been sick for quite some time as she had cancer in several parts of her body, and we ultimately knew her time was limited, but we weren't sure how long. She looked at me, and a tear began to bulge in my eye. She told me that she was going to be okay, but what she didn't necessarily realize was that I was not only crying about her. I was also crying due to the weight of the events that had happened right before I came to the hospital.

To her innocence, she even asked where Sophia was. I didn't know what to say. Do I spill the beans about what happened already, in front of several family members? Or do I just deflect and say that I already dropped her off before I got the call?

I settled with the second option for the moment because I didn't know what was going on myself. How could I tell my extremely sick grandmother what had happened? She needed nothing but positivity from everyone in the room, and I wasn't going to be the one to ruin that … not yet, at least.

That night finally ended. I laid in my own bed, but sleep eluded me for obvious reasons. My mind was racing. *How was my grandma? Do I still have a girlfriend? I can't talk to anyone about what's all on my mind because I don't want my family's attention to be away from my grandma.* These thoughts raced through my mind.

I finally fell asleep and woke up the next morning in a very apathetic mood. I just wanted to be alone. I didn't want to talk to anyone, and I am not a person that likes to talk about my feelings because I'd rather not have their pity. I don't want to be the center of attention or feel like I'm making my problems out to be worse than what others are going through.

I spent most of the day moping around the house. My mom asked if I was okay; I just said that I was sad thinking about grandma, which was obviously true. I was sad thinking about her and how devastated my Grandpa Alvin, my Grandma Cheryl's husband, must be feeling. However, that was obviously only half the reason for my state of mind.

Not much else happened for the rest of the week as I just tried to focus on working and getting ready to go back to school. The only thing worth noting about the rest of this week is that several people, such as my father, sister Celeste, and a few of my co-workers, were noticing a change in my mood. I wasn't being mean or anything; they just told me that I seemed "different" or "distracted." But as I said, I still didn't want to acknowledge what I was going through.

Spring Break ended, and I went back to school for the rest of the semester. Over the next several weeks, I tried incessantly to contact Sophia, but she was almost completely unresponsive. At that point, I had no idea what the status of our relationship was, but I knew it wasn't good. Meanwhile, I tried to see my grandma in the hospital at least twice per week as I wasn't sure how much longer these visitations would last. However, I was positive I wanted to make the most of the time I had left.

CHAPTER 2: THUMBS UP

It was then mid-March 2016. I'd been frequently visiting my grandma in the hospital, but my family, including her, was noticing that Sophia and I weren't really seeing each other. They began asking where she was. I had been deflecting for a while by saying she was busy with school, but I finally had enough of avoiding the question. She wasn't contacting me to see how I was doing. She wasn't asking how my grandma was. She wasn't doing anything that someone who cares would do, so I finally crumbled. I couldn't hold it in any longer.

My grandma asked me why Sophia had never come to visit her, and with a tear running down my face, I told my grandma that I didn't think we were together anymore because she wanted some time to herself to figure out her life.

Everyone in the room seemed shocked. I think they somewhat expected this, but hearing it come out of my mouth was still surprising.

You know how they say that getting stuff off your chest makes you feel better? Yeah, that wasn't the case here. It felt final to me now. There was no "maybe" anymore. My family knew, and when your family knows these sorts of things, they become final. With that said, I felt like I let everyone down in the room; I usually was the strong one for everyone. Now, I wasn't. I was weak and vulnerable.

My mental health only proceeded to grow worse in the coming weeks. I began eating only 400 calories per day — I just wasn't hungry and felt that losing weight would make me feel better about myself.

The caveat to that is that you can lose weight and love your physical image, but that will never make your mind or heart feel better. That's where your health actually starts. It starts in your heart and your mind. You have to be happy to love what you see in the mirror.

I knew I needed to get help. My mom helped me find a psychologist nearby that I went to once a week, and I'll be honest, it did help. Having someone to tell my full story to without having to omit details due to the anonymity was relieving. Despite this, I still had no appetite, which was VERY rare for me as I am usually a person who can eat a lot.

I saw the psychologist for a few weeks, and my grandma had been moved to a hospice as the doctors didn't think she had very long to live. It was late March, and I had an appointment one afternoon. As soon as I walked into the psychologist's office, I received a call from my dad; but he knew I was there, so why was he calling? I figured I'd let it go and call him back after my appointment. That was until he called again. I knew something had to have been going on because my dad wouldn't call again unless he needed to get ahold of me. I told the psychologist that I was going to take the call really quick.

This was not the call that I wanted. My dad told me that my grandma might only have 2 hours left to live according to the doctors. Everything in me dropped to the floor, and my expression went blank. I didn't know what to say. He said "Bub, you there?" Bub was a common nickname for me in my family. I said, "Yeah … sorry. I'm going to tell the psychologist that I'll have to reschedule." She understood the circumstances, and I left to go to the hospice to see my grandma for what I thought was the last time.

I arrived, but not before I cried the whole ride there. The combination of the end of my grandma's life along with presumably seeing my grandpa's distress was hard to swallow. I walked into my grandma's room, and probably thirty people or so were crammed inside trying to say their presumed goodbyes.

I noticed that my grandpa was not in the room, which was strange to me. He was always right by my grandma's side, so why was he not in the room at that moment? I found him sitting alone with his head down in a lounge room down the hallway from my grandma's room, and I knew this was about to be rough. I sat down next to him and put my arm around his shoulders. I told him I was always there if he needed me just like I know he'd be there if I needed him.

He had a small smirk go across his face despite the tear rolling down his cheek. He looked at me and said, "You know, Bub... you don't have to be strong for any of us. I know what you're going through isn't easy, either. We are a family; we look out for each other in tough situations."

That hit hard. I instantly began to get emotional. It was literally exactly what I wanted someone to say to me. I had been trying so hard to keep it together for everyone else that I lost sight of the fact that it's okay to not always be okay. You don't have to always be the hero in the story. Sometimes, even heroes need saving.

I think what made this moment so impactful was that my grandpa was not usually an emotional guy. He was by no means a "hard" man; he just wasn't one for crying or showing weakness in front of people. Seeing him in a state of vulnerability was abnormal to me as he wasn't one to show this side very often. He was only one to cry when truly in pain, so his tears implied so much more emotion than a regular person.

My grandpa and grandma had been together over forty years at that point, and they were genuinely ALWAYS together. They'd spent literally two-thirds of their lives together, so I couldn't fathom thinking about what it must be like to build a life with someone and see them in such agonizing pain.

We mutually agreed to walk back into my grandma's room to see everyone, and that's when I had my moment of realizing this was it. An entire lifetime of memories of my grandma flooded my mind. All the camping trips from my youth that my sister and I would go on with our grandparents, all the ball games that my grandma would be the loudest person cheering at, all the times that she would mediate family disagreements … All of it came rushing at me, and it was one of those moments that everything around me was drowned out. I couldn't really hear anything, and it seemed like I was secluded in darkness. I had to snap out of it quickly, though, with the mood in the room so somber that I didn't feel like adding to it.

My mom, dad, sister, Uncle Todd (my mom's brother), and I stayed there that night until the visiting hours ended. My grandpa had been staying in the hospice room with my grandma for her entire duration there, which normally isn't allowed, but he received special permission to do so. My grandma was unable to talk a whole lot, so she didn't actually say "goodbye" to us, but she loved communicating by giving people a thumbs up. The reason for this? I'm not entirely sure to this day, but it's what she did, so it caught on, and we all went along with it. We all gave her a thumbs up as we walked out, and she returned the favor.

Surprisingly, my grandma didn't pass away that night, but something felt different afterwards. Much like my relationship with Sophia, something about seeing my grandma the night before felt final, and even though she was still alive, it felt like the process of saying my official goodbyes had truly begun. Obviously, I knew for quite some time that she wasn't doing well, but that moment in her room with everyone let me know her time was close.

CHAPTER 3: WHEN IT RAINS, IT POURS

I just wanted to be alone. I needed to think. I felt that if I was around people, they'd know I was in pain, and, as was the usual with me, I didn't like that. I don't like being the center of attention, and I don't like people pitying me. I wanted to lose myself in something, so I went out to the movies … alone. And when I say "alone," I mean alone. I saw a movie called "Eddie the Eagle" without a single other person in the theater. The movie was about a young boy with a disability and a goal of being an Olympic ski jumper. Eddie was reminded constantly that he wouldn't be able to be what he wanted, but he kept trying anyways.

With no intent to spoil the film, there was a part of the movie where Eddie met a former Olympic ski jumper that he convinced to mentor him. He told the coach that he wanted to go on the second largest ski jump at the practice facility. His coach laughed at him and told him that it wasn't smart for a beginner to do that. Eddie didn't let that stop him from giving it a try.

As expected, he went up the second biggest hill and did not successfully land when he came down. In fact, he injured himself and almost couldn't participate in the qualifying jump to get into the Olympics. To qualify for the Olympics, Eddie had to hit a fabricated minimum distance that was determined by his country's Olympic board. They gave him a minimum distance that he had to jump before they'd recognize him as an Olympian. Long story short, during his qualifying jump, he ended up meeting the requirement, so they had no choice but to recognize him as an Olympian.

Watching this movie meant a lot to me at that moment. I needed some motivation and knowing that no matter how many times in life you get knocked down, you have to get back up on your feet. It sounds cliché, I know, but it's true.

If you don't get back up every time you fall, Life is going to keep running you over without mercy. You have to stand tall and have hope. You are never defeated until you lose hope.

I tried to keep this mindset for the time going forward. That is, until the morning of April 8th. I woke up at 5:00 AM to the sound of my mom screaming. It startled me so much that I really didn't know what to do. She was crying and screaming at the same time, so I knew something was obviously wrong, and I had a feeling of what it was.

Unfortunately, my feeling was correct. My dad was holding my mom, and I asked what was wrong. He told me that my grandma had passed away. No matter how much you prepare yourself for moments like these, they always come as a shock. I asked my dad if I should email my college professors to let them know that I wouldn't be in class for the day, but he told me to go ahead and go to class if I'd like since my grandma's room would be crowded. I decided that going to school could possibly be a necessary distraction from dealing with mourning my grandma.

I decided to lay back down in bed since I didn't need to be at school for a couple more hours and I wanted the sleep, but I had a really sharp pain in my side, which prevented me from getting the rest I needed. I finally fell back asleep and woke up around 8:30. I had class at 10:00, and it was only a half-hour drive, so that was fine.

When I woke up, that pain in my side had intensified quite a bit. I was thinking that perhaps I needed to use the restroom, or I just slept on my side in a funny way. I pondered staying home from school, but I decided to leave just because I wanted to mentally escape. Plus, I had to pick up my best friend Caleb because we carpooled to school, and it was my turn to drive. My mom and dad had left to go to the hospice to support my grandpa.

I left to pick up Caleb around 9:15, and the pain in my side was intense. I got to Caleb's house, which was only about 2 minutes away from my house, and he got in my car. I told him about my grandma and how I just wanted to go to school to get my mind off things. We pulled out of his driveway, and I began driving to school. I only made it about a mile down the road when my vision became extremely blurry. The pain in my side had become so strong that I was literally blacking out.

I immediately pulled over into a Speedway parking lot and parked. I was lucky that I could see enough to do that. I told Caleb that I couldn't see and that I had an extreme pain in my side. We mutually agreed that it was best that I didn't go to school. He offered to drive me to the hospital, but I told him if I sat there for just a minute, I'd be okay to drive him back home, so he could go to school since it wasn't far. To prevent him from worrying, I told him I was going to call the ambulance, so I would have a professional with me in case something went haywire.

I dropped him off and made my way home. The pain was intensifying by the minute. I parked my car and looked at our driveway, which was somewhat steep, so I was dreading the walk up it. I got out of my car, and I couldn't even stand up fully. I struggled up the driveway and stumbled into the house. I immediately fell on the floor and curled in a ball. I was always known for having a good pain tolerance, so when I say that this hurt, it hurt.

I called my mom and let her know that I didn't go to school and that I was having this awful pain in my side. I originally was going to wait for them to get home to call the ambulance, but I knew that she and my dad were at the hospice together, and I felt that I needed help immediately. My mom told me that they wouldn't be able to be home for roughly 45 minutes if they left right away. For a moment, I thought I was okay with that.

However, once I was off the phone with my mom, I knew that waiting 45 minutes on top of a probable half-hour drive to the hospital and a wait in the waiting room wasn't going to suffice with this pain. I needed to go now. I called the ambulance, and they said that they'd be at my house in roughly 10 minutes. In the meantime, I called my mom back and told her that I was going straight to the hospital. I wasn't able to wait that long, and she understood.

I felt so bad for this. Much like the situation with Sophia, I felt like I was taking away from the situation with my grandma. I just knew that I needed to get this checked out. This pain wasn't normal. This very easily could have gotten me in a car wreck earlier. I kept internally having an argument with myself on the way to the hospital. One side of me was thinking "Are you dumb? This pain is unreal." The other side of me was like "Everyone is probably thinking you want all the attention on you." I eventually settled with the justification that my grandma would want me to get myself checked out. I knew that's what she would have wanted me to do, so I found solace in that.

I finally arrived at the hospital with the medics that drove me, and surprisingly, my parents arrived not too long after, which made sense because the hospice wasn't all that far from the hospital. Doctors were coming in and out, and after repeatedly being asked my name and birthday, they decided to run some tests on me. They did a physical examination and took some X-rays. I sat in the room for quite a while with my parents. Surprisingly, Sophia tried calling me. She was presumably calling because she heard about my grandma. I'm not sure if that was the reason though; I just assumed it was. I ignored the call because I just honestly wasn't in the mood to talk to her. It was convenient that she called right when my grandma passed away to make it look like she cared about the state that I was in. Even if that wasn't the case, that's how it felt.

After a long wait, the doctors came into the room and told me that they thought that I was just backed up and needed to make some bowel movements. I thought that this conclusion seemed a bit off because I just didn't think needing to use the restroom could possibly cause this much pain. But they were the doctors, so I took their advice. They wrote me a prescription for some pain medicine and a laxative to try to relieve my issue.

I went home with my parents afterward still having the sharp pain in my side. I tried to ignore it and convince myself that the prescription would help me. We went ahead and dropped off the prescription to be filled at the local pharmacy near our house to be picked up later that day.

A lot of family and friends were going over to my grandparents' house that evening to be together and be there for my grandpa. We all hung out for a bit, and despite the tension of my grandma's passing lingering over the room, everyone was generally happy to be there for each other.

After being with everyone for an hour or so, my mom and I went back up to the pharmacy to get my prescription and went back to my grandparents' house. I had to drink this absolutely revolting cherry-flavored Magnesium Citrate drink to cause me to make bowel movements. The thought of it makes me sick to this day.

It took me 2 hours to drink this nausea-inducing drink. Every sip made me want to hurl, but I finally finished it, and I decided to head home at that point so that people didn't have to see me going to the restroom multiple times in a row.

I spent the next day-and-a-half in the restroom, but I was still having that awful pain in my side. I told myself that if the pain persisted into the next day that I was going back to the hospital to be re-evaluated. Something about the first diagnosis seemed wrong the whole time, so I just settled with that mindset.

Just to be safe, I called my boss to let her know everything that was going on and that I wouldn't be able to work that weekend. She understood, and I was able to find someone to pick up my shifts. I also emailed my professors at school to let them know I wouldn't be in class the rest of the week, but I'd only be missing 2 days of school since I didn't go every day. The only class that I missed anything in was Philosophy, which had daily small-value quizzes, but I figured that my situation was justification for missing a couple days.

CHAPTER 4 : PAIN, PAIN GO AWAY

I woke up in the morning with the pain persisting in my side. It was almost as bad as it was the morning before. I told my mom that I didn't think the doctors got my diagnosis correct because I had plenty of bowel movements the day before, and I was still having severe pain. She understood, and I asked her to take me back to the hospital.

We arrived at the hospital, and every bump in the road on the way made me cringe. It felt like someone was stabbing me right beneath the rib cage. We sat in the waiting room for someone to call us back, which always takes way longer than it should. In the meantime, my mom called my dad to update him that we had went back to the hospital because I was still in a lot of pain.

We finally had a doctor make his way out to have me come back into a room with him. He had me explain what was going on, so I told him the story of how I had been there the previous day but that I felt that I was not properly diagnosed since I was still in pain. He listened, said he wanted to look at my chart, and ordered a new X-ray of my kidneys.

Sitting at the hospital in pain is not fun, and it felt like I waited an eternity for someone to come back into my room to take me for this round of X-rays. I was just ready to know what actually was wrong with me. While waiting, my mom got a call from my dad asking how I was doing. He told both of us that he was going to try to finish his work early so that he could come see me.

As a small note, my dad is a mailman. He works hard and very rarely calls off, so if he tells his boss he needs to leave early, his boss is pretty lenient with him. My dad said he was going to try to get off around 3:30 that afternoon to head to the hospital since we all assumed that I'd be there for a while. Nothing is ever "fast" in a hospital.

A pair of nurses came into the room after a bit and took me to get the X-rays. I was afraid of what the result of the X-rays would be since I was already improperly diagnosed.

The nurses had me put on a protective vest that was made to block the potentially harmful rays, and they had me sit perpendicular to the X-ray machine so that they could get a shot of the side of my body. They also had me raise my arms vertically so that the bones in my arm didn't distort the view of my side. Needless to say, this wasn't very comfortable as stretching out in that manner only irritated the pain in my sides more.

The operator finished taking the X-rays, and the two nurses that brought me in picked me up to take me back to my original room. When we arrived back, my dad was sitting in the room with my mom. My mom had an uneasy look on her face, and I could almost read her mind as to what was bothering her.

My mom has always been a very dedicated family member. You really won't find someone that will do literally whatever they can to help the people they love quite like my mom.

With that level of connection, she is also cursed with feeling the pain of the people she cares about. If someone she loves is hurting, she'll be hurting just as much as they are.

With that in mind, I could only imagine that she was emotionally feeling the pain that I was going through from my situation with Sophia, my current medical situation, and the idea of her losing her mother (and both of her children losing their grandmother). I knew that had to be killing my mom internally just because of how much she connects herself to those she cares about.

My dad was always very good about comforting my mom in situations like this. My dad and I always had the same mentality that we always wanted to be the people that were strong for others when things were tough. It has never been a "macho" kind of tough. It's more of a "I'll always be there to be strong for you when you're weak" sort of tough.

I could only imagine my dad telling my mom that there was no way in the world he was going to let all of us hurt forever. He would never allow that, and that's always what I admired about my dad. I'm sure he was in pain as well watching his son lay there in the hospital bed and knowing that his wife just lost her mother, but my dad was always a symbol of consistency. If I've ever felt lost, my dad was always such a good person to go to.

I caught myself zoning out thinking about what emotions were going on in my parents' minds, but I snapped out of it when a doctor walked in with my X-ray results. As I said earlier, I was nervous. I had never felt pain like this before, and I hoped that it was nothing life-threatening. The doctor organized his stack of papers and opened his folder with my results in it.

He looked at me and told me that they found kidney stones deposited in my ureters on both sides of my body. I asked why I was only experiencing pain on one side then, and he told me that the stone on that side was the bigger of the two, and the stone on the other side hadn't begun moving quite yet. He said that this was obviously a much better explanation for the pain I was experiencing than being "backed up." I concurred with this assessment as I had heard from numerous people that kidney stones are incredibly painful. And word to the wise, if someone tells you that kidney stones hurt, they're not lying.

The doctor wrote me a prescription for Vicodin to help with my pain and referred me to a kidney specialist by the name of Dr. Ali. The doctor told me that in the meantime, I should drink a lot of water and try to be active because the more you move around, the more likely the stone was to move and hopefully come out. With that in mind, I told myself that I was going to begin running after my grandma's funeral in a couple days. I felt that I mentally and physically deserved a few days off with all that had been going on, but I knew that running would help take my mind off of all the thoughts racing through my mind.

We checked out of the hospital and made our way home. I was still in a fair amount of pain, but I was much more content with my diagnosis this time. Having kidney stones explained the pain so much better than basically being constipated. On the way home, I called my grandpa just to see how he was doing and asked if he needed anything. He usually was one to decline help from others, but he told me that he did have something he would like me to do. Before even asking what he needed, I agreed to help him because it was so rare for him to ask for something that there was no way I'd turn him down.

He asked me if I could speak at my grandma's funeral. I felt honored, and I felt that I had the opportunity to use my current situation to help other people get through my grandmother's passing. I spent the next four to five days preparing my grandmother's eulogy. I was given the option to read a generic eulogy, but I wanted to write this from my heart. I had too much to say to not take this opportunity.

The day before my grandma's funeral, Sophia sent me a text message saying that she heard about my grandmother and that she planned on attending the funeral. Great, just what I wanted… this was destined to be awkward. Was I supposed to act normal like nothing happened? Was I supposed to act like I was totally okay with her ignoring me for weeks and not being there for me when my grandmother was dying? Was I supposed to just be cordial and not let the rest of the people at the funeral know that we were no longer a thing? All I said in response to her text was "Thanks." That's all I was willing to say to her. She didn't deserve anything more than that at that point.

CHAPTER 5: BREATHE

The day of my grandmother's funeral had come. I had spent the better part of a week writing and perfecting what I was going to say. I had an important message to convey. Losing my grandma, being hospitalized, and being essentially abandoned by someone all at the same time had taken quite a toll on me, and I felt that what I said at the funeral could perhaps help someone else.

We arrived at the funeral an hour before the actual viewing because immediate family was allowed to share that time together before anyone else arrived. My grandpa looked completely heartbroken. But how couldn't he be? I felt utterly distraught from a relationship that ended after six years, so I couldn't imagine what it must feel like to be with someone for over forty years and lose them permanently. My grandma was his best friend, and he didn't have that anymore.

I'm a person who has self-diagnosed second-hand sadness. I'm more likely to cry from seeing someone else in pain than I am from my own personal pain. I could feel my grandpa's pain. I had to step out of the room; I just couldn't see him hurt like that.

I went outside and walked to my parents' car because I had forgotten the eulogy I had written for my grandma on the backseat. I didn't need to have the paper as I had it memorized. I just needed a reason to walk away from seeing my grandpa in so much pain.

I sat outside in the car for a few moments by myself. Sometimes, you just want to be alone. Sometimes, you just need to process things on your own to have personal clarity. I was having that feeling again. My sister and I would never see our grandmother again. My grandpa would never see his wife again. My mother and uncle would never see their mother again.

That's part of life, which is not meant to be eternal. It's not supposed to last forever because it would be way less special. If it lasted forever, people would value it even less than they already do. People have a very difficult time processing the end of anything, but death forces us to accept it as reality whether we like it or not.

As more people arrived, I figured it was time to make my way back inside and meet back up with my family. A lot of people knew my grandma. She had a vast assortment of friends, and we always had an inside joke within the family that she knew someone wherever we would go. She would find someone to talk to regardless of where she was. She had an infectious and outgoing personality, so it only made sense that she had a lot of people that cared about her.

A large crowd of people were in line waiting to pay their respects to my grandmother. All of the immediate family sat in the front, and people talked to us as they made their way to the front of the line. There were some people crying, there were some people catching up with others they hadn't seen in a while, and some people still trying to process what was going on.

I saw Sophia and her mother walk in the front door. I'll admit, I was a bit surprised she actually showed up. I had grown to not really put too much value to her "promises," so her being there was somewhat shocking. Her mother was holding a bouquet of flowers for my mom. I had no issue with anyone in Sophia's family. What happened between us was no fault of her family, so I thanked her mother for coming. As for Sophia, this was next-level awkward. What do I say? A number of sarcastic comments came to mind. I decided to be polite and give her a simple head nod and a "Thanks for coming." She could tell that I was being evasive, but I had nothing to say to her that would have been appropriate at this time of grieving. She sat down with others as the preacher began.

The preacher's name was Jimmy. He had been a friend of the family for longer than I'd been alive. I'll be honest, I didn't know his last name; he might even be related to me. Everyone always just called him "Jimmy," so I went along with it. He told his story of how he knew my grandparents and shared fond memories of them, which brightened the mood in the room. This was a good start.

My father then read the obituary. My sister followed him, and she spoke about my grandma and how she knows that even though my grandma will miss physical events in her grandkids' lives, she will be there in spirit and that she will have the best view of everyone.

It was then my turn to speak. I looked out at everyone in the crowd and tried to fight back a tear that I knew would come out at some point. I glanced at my paper and didn't look at it again because the words came from my heart.

> *Today is a day that celebrates the life of a wonderful person. Sure, we all already miss her, but an important message can be learned from my grandmother's life. For those of you that knew the situation of the days leading up to her passing, you knew that she struggled greatly to breathe.*
>
> *Being able to breathe is a blessing. I think there are many moments throughout our lives where people forget how much they have to be thankful for. Has anyone here ever taken the time to appreciate breathing? It's something our bodies do naturally, but we don't even consciously think about it. It keeps us alive, but we never take the time to appreciate it.*
>
> *On that note, I have a metaphor for you all. I call it 'The Metaphor of the Tree.' You may be wondering what this is. Well, I will start with a question. Much like I asked earlier, does everyone here realize that trees supply our oxygen for us to breathe? Without trees, we literally couldn't survive. Yet, I would venture as far to say that most people in this room, if not every person in this room, have never felt appreciative of what trees do for us.*

You're probably now wondering what my point is. Well, my point is that so much goes into our lives, and so many things occur naturally that are necessary for us to live that occur without us having to do anything. Our brain creates all our thoughts and conducts our whole bodies. Our heart pumps blood so that it functions properly. Our legs move with ease so that we can get from place to place. Yet we don't appreciate them until these things can no longer operate on their own.

I don't think it is a mystery that my grandma would have loved to breathe on her own in her last days, but she had to have oxygen pumped into her lungs. My message to every person in this room today is to appreciate what you have. Appreciate the little things before you lose them. They say that you don't know what you've got until it's gone. Change that. Know what you have. Love and cherish what you have before it is gone. Without having to ask her, I'm sure my grandma would say the same thing. Thank you and rest in peace, Grandma.

As I walked away from the podium, I gave a thumbs up towards the sky. I knew that not everyone in the room knew what that meant, but that was okay. I knew what it meant, and that's all that mattered.

I could tell that my speech had really affected some people in the crowd. Plenty of people were crying in their seats. My goal wasn't to make people cry. I just wanted people to appreciate things before it was too late. I hoped my message sank in.

The speeches had concluded, and people began making their way to the front to give their condolences to my family. The pallbearers then carried my grandmother's coffin outside to the hearse that would transport her to the cemetery. I wasn't actually able to carry her coffin due to my kidney stones, so I followed others out.

CHAPTER 6: THE MOMENT OF TRUTH

It was time to head to the cemetery to truly say goodbye to my grandmother. A long line of cars with small purple flags drove down Interstate 35, one after the other. The cemetery where my grandmother was to be buried was 20 minutes away, yet the drive felt as if it took hours. The car was quiet since no one was in the mood to listen to music or talk. The only noise that could be heard was the constant spin of tires against the pavement.

This lack of noise was somewhat of a hint at what the near future would hold: silence. Some situations are beyond words. Sometimes, there just isn't a right thing to say, so silence is the only clear choice.

The long and quiet ride came to an end at the entrance to the cemetery. Rows upon rows of tombstones lined the grass. I'm not sure how most people feel, but when I look at tombstones or gravesites, I can't help but wonder what the people buried beneath were like. What struggles did they face during their lives? Were they happy? What did they experience that I wasn't alive to experience?

I became reflective, thinking about how precious life is and what we do while on this earth. We were instructed to pull around to where my grandmother's plot was. The long line of cars snaked through the cemetery behind us.

Car after car stopped, and the crowd of people migrated to my grandma's grave. The pallbearers carried the casket from the hearse to the tent that was set up above the grave. A light, drizzling rain forced everyone to huddle closely to stay dry. Even though the temperature wasn't particularly cold that afternoon, no one felt "warm."

Jimmy began speaking again by leading with a prayer. Slight whispers of sobbing could be heard coming from the several dozen people gathered around. The sobbing combined with the light drizzling rain was a perfect combination to describe the mood: sadness. As I said, death is a finite idea. It is the end. I'd like to think that there is a wonderful afterlife to be lived, but death is a finite end to life on Earth.

Jimmy asked if anyone had anything to add to his prayer before the casket was lowered into the grave. Everyone remained silent. I don't believe anyone was in the mood to talk. I know I wasn't. I had spoken my peace earlier, and I had nothing more to say.

Several people pulled flowers from the bouquet that rested on top of the casket as a final reminder of the life that had ended. Once everyone that wanted a flower had grabbed theirs, the casket was lowered into the damp ground, and it was official — my grandmother was now eternally resting.

Everyone began walking back to their cars when Sophia sent me a text message to come over to her car for just a minute. What did she want? I had just watched my grandma be lowered into the grave. I didn't want any additional drama, but I reluctantly walked to Sophia's car. Her mom was sitting in the passenger seat, and Sophia was leaning up against the car.

I had a blank look on my face. I was in a very somber mood for obvious reasons. She said, "Sorry for what you had to go through today." I remained silent as I nodded my head as a subtle hint of acknowledgement. I asked, "Was there anything you needed to tell me, or was that it?" I could tell that she was keeping something from me by the distant look in her eyes, but I didn't want to get into that discussion now. It wasn't the right time.

After a moment of awkward silence, she motioned toward me as if she was going to give me a sympathy hug. I backed away and said that I needed to go because everyone was heading over to my Uncle

Terry's, my grandma's uncle, for lunch and to spend time together. She nodded with a look of disappointment. Oh well. I just didn't need any more negative energy, and I knew that continuing the conversation with her could lead to that. I felt as if I was being a little cold, but I had the right to be. Sophia and I were together for six years, and she both physically and emotionally abandoned me when I needed her the most.

I proceeded to make my way to the car. The line was now exiting the cemetery, and each vehicle either headed home or began making the short trip to my Uncle Terry's house. Uncle Terry's house was only 5-10 minutes from the cemetery, so we arrived there quickly.

Quite a crowd had already congregated at my uncle's house. My Aunt Carol, Terry's wife, had begun preparing food, and there were tables set up outside. Luckily, the rain had stopped, and the sun was starting to show a bit, so we were able to gather outside. I saw a basketball hoop in the driveway and started throwing up a couple of shots.

A few people joined in shooting around waiting for the food. My cousins Johnny, Jordan, Couper, my Uncle Todd, my dad, and I were all messing around on the small makeshift court. It was nice to have a little fun on such an emotionally dark day. I was especially happy to see Todd trying to have a good time with us since he just had to bury his mom. There was no way that wasn't hard for him.

We were shooting for about a half-hour when Aunt Carol yelled out to everyone that the food was ready. It had already been a long day, and I'm sure everyone was hungry. Being able to eat all together was good for everyone as it allowed each of us to mentally escape from the loss of my grandma for a short period of time.

We were all gathered around a picnic table when, all of a sudden, I received a call from Sophia. I walked away from the table and went to a secluded spot away from everyone because I had a weird feeling about why she was calling. I felt that this could be the long-awaited conversation.

"Hello?" I answered.

Sophia sounded a bit down when she asked, "What do you want me to do with your stuff?"

"I don't need it anytime soon. Drop it off whenever you can," I replied.

Awkward pause.

"Once again," Sophia said, "I'm sorry for your grandma."

"Thanks," I said while trying to be dismissive.

Another awkward pause.

"How are you so okay with this?" asked Sophia. "I figured you'd be way more down."

I was taken aback by her inquisition. Did she want me to be more down? Was she hoping that I was sad or upset?

"Well, what am I supposed to do?" I asked back. "I have to find a way to be happy somehow. I've had to face this alone, so I was already searching for a way to be happy."

I decided to start asking her questions.

"My question is, how are *you* so okay with this? I'm not really in the mood to fight or argue, but what have you been up to for the last two months?"

In my gut, I already felt I knew the answer to my question, but I wanted to hear it from her.

Sophia was hesitant to speak as she clearly wanted to choose her words wisely.

"Well, I had been talking to Jeremy, and …" she began.

I knew where this was going. Jeremy was a friend of her sister's boyfriend. Sophia's sister and her boyfriend lived together, and Jeremy often hung out with them. It was beginning to make sense why Sophia would always want to go hang out with her sister and why I was never invited.

"Jeremy understands me so well," Sophia continued, "and you and I had been arguing so much. He and I just really connected."

I had a bevy of snappy comebacks to say to that, but I instead just asked, "How long was this going on?"

I had known that Sophia had been talking to Jeremy since at least winter. I went over to her mom's house to see her one night, and when I walked in the door, her phone was lying on the couch. It vibrated, and I briefly glanced at it and saw Jeremy's name pop up. I didn't read the message, but I made a mental note of it. I asked her about it later, and she gave me the typical, "Oh, it's nothing for you to worry about." I still had a feeling it was something to worry about despite her "assurance."

A moment of silence passed. Sophia was presumably deciding between lying and telling the truth. She then continued, "Well, we had begun talking in the winter, and our conversations were usually always about you and I at first. I just wanted someone to talk to about our problems, but I didn't want to bring them up to you because I was afraid that you'd get mad."

I made a really dumb look on my face and I, very sarcastically, retorted, "Oh, so you were worried about me being mad, but you didn't think that confiding in another guy would make me upset. Good logic."

Sophia had to have known I was triggered by this point. I asked, "So what have you been doing with him the last two months while you were ignoring my existence?"

I was becoming snappier with my jabs, and I could tell it was affecting her. She paused again. "I have been staying with him at his place."

"Whoa … *staying* with him?" I asked, dumbfounded.

To be honest, I had been suspicious of this. I was just more surprised that she was being so honest with me. I only had one question left to ask, and I already knew the answer, but I wanted to hear her admit it. "Did you sleep with him?"

It was very apparent she didn't want to answer this. She knew that her answer would be incriminating.

She avoided the question temporarily and asked, "Is there ever a chance for us in the future if he and I don't work out?"

I, once again appalled at her logic, decided to state, "You didn't answer my question."

Clearly searching for what to say, she hesitantly spoke, "We got drunk, and it progressed from there."

I already assumed this was the case; I wasn't stupid. I just wanted her to say it. Now, I knew just what to say in return.

"To answer your question, hell no. We are done ... permanently. I was done with you before I knew this because of how you abandoned me," I said. "This was just more confirmation that my thought process was correct. Have a nice life. I hope you two work out just fine."

I obviously was not being sincere. I didn't mean that last statement in the slightest. I heard her begin to speak, but I hung up the phone. She tried to call back immediately, but I declined the call.

That was the last time I ever spoke to Sophia. I didn't need that. I deserved so much more than what she gave. I'll be the first to admit I'm not perfect. I've made my mistakes. I made plenty of mistakes in my relationship with Sophia. I'm not ashamed to admit that, but I knew I deserved someone who was willing to reciprocate the effort that I put in. She clearly wasn't that person.

I will admit it did hurt, though. It wasn't necessarily the fact that I lost her that hurt. What hurt was the aftermath. The self-questioning that would soon ensue. The pain of wondering what I did to deserve that, the feeling of not being enough, of being alone when I desperately wanted someone to confide in, the feeling of being replaced. These thoughts were what hurt the most.

CHAPTER 7: PROMISES MADE

Sheesh, what a day. What a week, honestly. Let's recap... I got kidney stones, and my grandma passed away on the same day. Then, a few days later, I had my grandmother's funeral, and I found out that Sophia had been cheating on me. I had already made a promise to myself that I was going to start exercising and running after my grandma's funeral, so I figured that I might as well start that night. I decided that I was going to go running once we left my Uncle Terry's house.

After the conversation with Sophia, I walked back over to my family who was still gathered around the picnic tables. My mom and dad simultaneously asked who called me. I told them that I would tell them later. I felt that it wasn't the time or place for it. I didn't want the attention to be on me and definitely not for that reason. Celeste overheard the conversation as she was sitting nearby. I want to be very clear about this: nothing is ever subtle with my sister. I don't mean that in a bad way; she just isn't a person to let something go unconfronted.

She pulled me aside and said, "Let's talk." Since we would be away from everyone, I didn't mind telling her. I told her the full story, and with no exaggeration; she was LIVID. My sister, despite being younger than me, always had a self-imposed mission to defend me. She has always been a protective younger sibling. It isn't common, I know, but it is the truth. She has had her moments of being a pain in my butt like any younger sister, but she truly is a great one. She has always looked up to me, so I have always taken pride in being a good older brother and role model.

I won't go into details, but let's just say, she wasn't particularly happy with Sophia. She used some much more colorful language than I should say, but, like I said, she was *not* happy.

My sister then said, "Hey, you know what we should do?"

"What?" I responded.

"We should go get some ice cream or something and go on a drive tonight. Just drive around and get our minds off today."

I agreed that her plan sounded fun. Plus, I didn't mind having something to do in between my uncle's house and going on my run later that night.

We walked back over to join the family again, and our parents asked if everything was okay. I was still insistent that I would tell them later as I just wanted to spend time with the family.

My family and I left late that afternoon to head home. I told my parents what had happened on the way. They both felt bad for me, but I told them that I was strangely a little relieved. I finally understood Sophia's actions to some degree. I no longer had to wonder what was going on. I had some closure. I told them that it hurt obviously, but I was still somehow relieved.

I didn't want to make a big deal of it. I kind of just wanted the day to be over. It had been a long one already, but, in a way, it was a day of resolution. It was a day of closure. That day brought finality. With every ending, starts a new beginning.

Once we got home, my sister and I changed and left again. We went to Sonic for drinks and to Wal-Mart to walk around. We didn't do anything special except be there for one another. We drove around listening to music at full blast playing goofy songs that made us laugh. We then headed home.

When we arrived, mom and dad told me that if I needed to talk, they would listen. They told me that I didn't need to minimize my feelings for any reason. I had a lot of reason to hurt, so I shouldn't suppress it. I declined for the moment just because I didn't want to think about it anymore. I was mentally done with that day. I didn't really want to think anymore.

Once it started getting dark that night, I told everyone that I was heading out for a run. It was strange, but I was excited to clear my mind. I created a music playlist suited for my mood, placed my phone in my running armband, and started jogging around town.

It was the first time I had ran in quite some time, so I could tell I was a bit out of shape. After roughly 15 minutes, I arrived at the local baseball field. Even though it rained during the day, it was a clear night. I wanted to sit in the bleachers looking out over the field under the stars to process all that had happened.

I'll preface that what I'm about to say sounds weird, but it's true. I always enjoyed having conversations with myself when I'm alone. The more I'm alone, the more philosophical my thoughts are. I guess, it's more like I just think out loud as opposed to "talking to myself."

I recollected on the events of the day, thinking about life and the lessons I learned from what had transpired. I made a mental note of what I wanted out of a relationship assuming I would be in another one at some point. I made myself a promise that I would never let myself get treated like an option again.

I promised myself that I would find someone that appreciates me the way that I would appreciate them. I promised that I would not give up on the possibility of loving again just because I had been betrayed once. I promised myself that I would never question myself and wonder if I was enough because I knew that I was. I knew that someone out in the world would appreciate what I had to offer.

I also promised myself to always appreciate the little things, such as breathing and all things in life that allow us to live and don't get enough credit. Basically, I reminded myself of what I said at the funeral. I would not let the past week defeat me and make me give up hope. In life, you cannot be defeated if you have hope.

I sat there in silence for quite some time just looking up at the night sky. It was beautiful. Looking at the night sky is so humbling. It makes you realize that the universe is so immense, incomprehensibly large, and impossible to quantify. It has that effect on me.

When I look at the night sky and the stars, it makes me feel like my problems, much like myself, are so small in comparison to the universe. And much like the effect of laughter, minimizing your issues always makes them easier to overcome.

I had hope for a brighter future. Don't get me wrong, I knew that darkness could come at any minute, but I had hope that things would get better. They had to. Things had to get better because this wasn't the end of my story.

I looked at my phone and realized that it was almost midnight. My mom had texted me twice asking where I was because I had been out for almost 2 hours. With that said, I exited the bleachers and started jogging home. I took the short way, which would only take five minutes or so if I jogged at a decent pace.

I probably pushed myself a bit too hard on the run home because I was very winded when I got in the door. I was a bit more winded than I should have been, but I attributed it to the fact that I ran at a pretty good pace, and I still wasn't in good running shape. I figured this would improve over time.

My mom was insistent again in telling me that I could talk to her about anything. I knew this was true, but I wasn't really wanting to talk about anything. I felt that I had a good mindset going forward. Make no mistake about it, I felt sad. I felt defeated. I felt as if I had been knocked down and kicked while I was there. But I knew internally that I wasn't going to give up hope no matter what happened. That was the only mindset I could have given the situation.

CHAPTER 8: DON'T LET ME MISS YOU

I had to return to school the following week for finals. I wasn't all that worried about the testing to be honest because I had retained really good grades despite all of my personal issues. At the end of the semester, I had 4 A's and a C. Normally, I would freak out over having a C, but I cut myself some slack considering all that I'd been through during the semester up to that point.

Despite having success in school and now being on summer break, I wasn't nearly as positive or upbeat as I normally would be. I really started to feel the after-effects of all that had happened.

I was going up to the track every night to get a few laps in and sit there alone thinking. You wouldn't believe how your mind wanders when there is almost complete silence and darkness.

In a way, it was almost like running at night took away my senses and forced me to understand what was going on inside of myself. I had to teach myself that everything was going to be okay from within. I had to rewire how my brain processed adversity.

Secluding myself from the outside world caused a lot of emotions to be exposed. Sometimes, I sat there and cried. Sometimes, I sat there pondering what the purpose of humanity was. Sometimes, I would run a lap at a full sprint and just scream at the top of my lungs just to prove to myself that I could push myself to the limits. I wasn't even afraid if anyone heard my screams or my sobbing because I was so cut off from the outside world.

I did this on purpose. I was running in the dark for a reason. It was almost like a personal metaphor to myself. I convinced myself that the symbolism of me running in the dark would equate to appreciating what I had in the light. I was using this as a method to show myself that no matter how many reasons I could find to give up, I could always find reasons not to. If I kept running in the dark, I would eventually appreciate the good things even more.

I would be lying if I said that there weren't times that I was at the track by myself wondering what the world would be like without me in it. I wasn't necessarily contemplating suicide or harming myself, but I did genuinely think of what me ceasing to exist would mean from an external point of view.

What mainly kept me from getting too close to "the ledge" was thinking about the people that would be affected if I were to give up. A promise that my mother and I had made to each other came to the forefront of my mind.

When I was younger, my mother and sister would have arguments all the time. They never got physically violent, but they were often very volatile towards one another. My sister would throw verbal jabs, and my mom would usually return the favor. There were times they both added fuel to the flame, but their disputes usually ended in one of them saying something way below the belt that would cause the other to completely shut down or even leave the house.

There were multiple times when my sister would just rush out of the front door and start running down the street. I usually was the one to go after her. I often felt she left just to see if anyone would search for her, almost to see if someone cared enough to come get her.

There were also multiple times when my mom would leave the house upset and just start driving. It's never a smart thing to drive while overly emotional. There is always a chance that something doesn't end well.

The promise that I mentioned was created one day when my mom and sister got into a big dispute, and my mom went on one of her emotional car drives. I wasn't home at the time; I was helping Sophia's dad power-wash their back porch that day, but I got a call from my mom. She had explained the dispute that she and my sister had and explained that she had been away from the house for several hours, and no one checked on her.

I had no idea as I hadn't been home for a decent amount of time. I asked her where she was several times and told her that I was coming to see her. I hate whenever I know someone feels alone in the manner that they believe that no one cares about how they are.

After several times of asking, I finally got my mom to tell me where she was, and I met her there. She had been sitting in a gazebo at a local park in Englewood for hours all by herself. I told her that I would get some ice cream, so we could eat it together.

She told me that sometimes she felt that it would be better if she weren't here. I told her that under no circumstance was that the case. There are always reasons to keep fighting. I told her that even if she and my sister fight, my sister would never be able to operate without her. I told her I needed her for so many things that I had yet to experience and that I always appreciate all that she does. I told her that my dad expects her to be his life partner. They were going to need each other especially once my sister and I move out.

At the end of me explaining all of this to her, she understood her place in the world. We were her place in the world. This is when I made her promise to never let me miss her. I made her the same promise to never let her miss me.

With that in mind, I couldn't let my mom miss me. I made a promise, and I had to abide by that. So even though I felt lost and confused, I had to find myself. I had to search through the darkness until I found the light inside of myself.

As for my dad, he always taught my sister and I to be fighters in life. By "fighter" I don't mean getting in fist fights; I mean always striving to prevail. Fighting through tough situations is what my dad instilled in both of us. I couldn't give up. I'd let my dad down. I'd let myself down if I gave up. I had a future ahead of me. I had a life to live. I had reasons to live. I was halfway done with my college degree.

There's no way I could give up.

My sister always looked up to me. What kind of older brother and role model would I be to her if I let a few bumps in the road stop me from continuing my forward momentum? I couldn't set that example for her. I had to keep fighting to show her that she should keep fighting when things got rough.

What about my grandpa? He just lost his wife. I couldn't put him through losing a grandkid, too. That would be selfish of me. I had people to fight for. I had myself to fight for.

These are the thoughts that kept me from truly contemplating suicide or from giving up hope for a better future. That doesn't, by any stretch, mean that all my thoughts were rainbows and unicorns. I'd say that 99% of what was going through my head at the time was darkness, loneliness, and contemplating what my purpose was. But that remaining 1% was enough to push forward.

Just as I was sitting at the track with all these conflicting thoughts going through my head, I received a text from my good friend Dexter asking if I wanted to hang out with him and go running. I was happy about this because I desperately needed a friend to confide in at the time. It was easy to connect with Dexter because he was also in and out of a relationship with a girl that wasn't faithful to him. We agreed to meet up at the track the following night, so we could run together and just hang out.

Even though I didn't mind being alone at the track, it was nice having someone with a shared experience to be able to relate to. Dexter is one of the few guy friends that I can discuss my feelings without the conversation being awkward. A lot of people would assume that two guys talking about relationships wouldn't be a heartfelt discussion, but I knew that I would be able to have good conversations with Dexter because he wasn't a guy that was afraid to show his emotions for the people he cared about.

CHAPTER 9: GASPING FOR AIR

Dexter and I hung out every night for about a week or two. We didn't go running quite every night, but we would just hang at each other's houses and play video games or talk about our recent relationship history. It was just nice having someone to relate to and to not feel quite so lonely.

We had been friends for several years prior to that summer but being able to run at the track and hang out with him made us the closest we had ever been. I will eternally be grateful for him being there for me, and I will always return the favor if he ever needed it. That's what friends are for.

Dexter's motivation for exercising was a bit different from mine. He wanted to get in shape and train for the Air Force, and he was set to leave for Basic Training mid-July. This gave him a little under two months to get himself up to where he needed to be. Mine was totally personal and used as a distraction from all that was going on. Still, it was nice having someone there that I knew cared about my well-being.

There was, however, one night that Dexter was unable to hang out or go up to the track. I still decided to go because it had become a routine in my life at that point. It was second nature to run once it got dark outside.

Doing my normal routine, I tried to complete several laps. One lap around a regulation track is 400 meters. To keep a consistent pace, I would usually jog the first 300 meters and then sprint the last 100 just to challenge myself. For whatever reason, I was struggling to keep my breath more than normal.

What was strange was that I knew I should have been in decent enough shape to do the running I was doing because of the length of time that had passed since I had begun. I'd been doing it practically every night for almost a month and hadn't struggled quite this much before.

That's when the pain hit. I'd made it around the track a few times and then an extremely sharp stab struck me in the side. I fell to the ground in agony. I immediately assumed the pain was from kidney stones; it was a very similar sensation and almost in the exact same spot but just a little higher, closer to my ribcage. If this was kidney stones, why was I having so much trouble breathing?

I was on the ground practically gasping for air when I mustered up the strength to walk to my car. Thankfully, I had decided to drive up to the track that night instead of run. I knew there was no way I would have been able to walk or run home. I called my dad because I knew he was home and told him of the pain. He also assumed it was kidney stones, but we were both so puzzled as to why I was struggling to breathe.

I made the short three-minute drive home and struggled up the driveway ... again. It was eerily similar to the situation with kidney stones except I at least had someone home with me. I got to the door, and my dad helped me over to the couch.

I took one of the pain pills that I was prescribed for kidney stones and sat there for a while. My dad and I talked about what was going on until my mom and sister finally got home.

They both asked what was wrong, and I explained to them what had happened. At the time, my sister was going to school to be a nurse, and my mother had a decent background in health as well, so they both were immediately concerned about what I had told them. My sister has a pulse oximeter, which checks the amount of oxygen a person has when you put the small machine on your index finger. She told me that she was going to check my oxygen levels since I said I was struggling to breathe, and I was taking short, quick breaths.

She placed the machine on my fingers, and the reaction on her face alarmed me. Her eyes grew large, and she said, "I'm gonna check this again." She pulled the machine off me and made sure it was calibrated correctly. The anticipation of waiting for the reading was making her anxious. She had the exact same reaction as when she first checked it. She looked at my mom and declared, "He needs to go to the hospital, *now*!"

Confused and worried, my mom, dad, and I all simultaneously asked, "Why? What is the reading?"

My sister said, "Forest, your reading is a 78. A person your age should have no lower than a 97 at any moment. To put that in perspective, a 78 is what someone who is over sixty-years-old and has smoked their entire life would have. You obviously aren't sixty, and you don't smoke, so something is going seriously wrong with your lungs right now."

You know that feeling you get when you hear something that shocks you, and you don't know how to process what you're hearing? You get a warm, prickly sensation in your torso, and you have a slight hot flash? That was me in that moment. I didn't know how to process what she just said; I just knew it was not good. My dad broke me out of the trance and told everyone to gather some things to go to the hospital. My mom grabbed what I needed, so I didn't have to make any unnecessary movements.

I made my way out to the garage to get into my parents' car. I sat in the front seat, so I could lay the seat back on my way to the hospital. Everyone gathered in the car, and my dad started driving right away. I closed my eyes the entire ride. The pain in my ribs was still very sharp, and I had to mentally tell myself to not breathe too fast. I had to convince myself to breathe slowly because breathing too fast increased the pain. Breathing deep did not create any comfort, however. In fact, it hurt almost just as bad as breathing fast; I just knew that it probably wasn't the best to breathe fast and get myself worked up.

After a half-hour drive or so, we arrived at Good Samaritan Hospital in Dayton. My dad dropped my mom and I off at the Emergency Room entrance, so I could hopefully get to see a doctor or a nurse faster than waiting in a waiting room for who knows how long.

I was only waiting a couple minutes when a nurse called me back. I stood up but was only able to hunch over because of the pain. The nurse saw me struggling and asked if I would like a wheelchair. I wanted so badly to decline, but I figured that it was probably best, so I didn't have to walk across the waiting room looking like the Hunchback of Notre Dame.

The nurse asked me the typical questions that you get asked every time you're in the hospital. "What's your name? What is your birthday? What brings you here? Do you smoke or drink alcohol?" I answered all the questions and told her the story of what had happened. I explained that I was in the hospital about a month ago for kidney stones. She grinned at me and said, "Man, you've had it rough recently." My immediate thought was, "Man, if she only knew." Plenty had happened to make things rough, but I figured there was no point in spilling my life story to this nurse. I'm sure she hears stuff like that from patients all the time, so I didn't really feel like being that guy for the moment.

The nurse wheeled me back to an examination room where she checked my vitals, and she also checked my oxygen levels. She seemed just as shocked as my sister at the readings. My oxygen level had decreased to 76. I had lost another 2% since we left home. I tried not to freak out, but I also was thinking that at that rate, I would be down to critical levels rather quickly if I already wasn't.

The nurse told me that a doctor would be in shortly, and she left the room. So here I was in a hospital room waiting on a doctor to come in and see me … again. I couldn't help but think of the ironic message that life was sending me at this moment. Not long before, I had been emphasizing that we should all be appreciative of breathing and the small things that life blesses us with without us even noticing. I had stressed that point at my grandma's funeral, and yet here I lay in a hospital bed struggling to breathe.

Was this Life testing me to see if I really appreciated it? Was it making sure that I really meant what I said and not just saying something for a reaction? It was almost comically ironic. I already thought that I genuinely appreciated breathing, but apparently, I had been taking it for granted. I apparently only had empathy for people that struggled to breathe prior to that night. That night gave me sympathy for those that couldn't breathe. This was a harsh test to see if I really appreciated breathing, but I guess it's important to find a silver lining in negative situations. I could at least have something to back up my message now.

I sat in silence in the all-white, sterile room for a while. I'm not even sure that I thought about anything. Honestly, what was there to think about? My mind was tired of thinking. The doctor came in and broke the silence. He asked me the same generic questions that I'd answered earlier and was also surprised that I was having that much trouble breathing considering I never smoked. He told me that they were going to be doing X-rays on my chest to see what was going on.

I was told a nurse would come get me shortly to take me back to get my X-rays, and then he left the room. My parents and sister walked into the room just a few moments after he had left. My dad told me that he and my sister would be heading home for the night to sleep, but he would be coming back in the morning to see me because he had already called off work for the next day. I hugged them goodbye and asked my mom what she was doing.

This was kind of a dumb question because I knew she was going to stay with me. She always did. I knew my mom wouldn't let me be alone in there. To be honest, I don't know why I even asked. She had spent the night with my sister and I every time we were in the hospital before, so I knew that wasn't going to change for this stint.

I grinned at her with an appreciative look on my face. At least I didn't have to be in there alone all night. With the condition I was apparently in, it seemed evident that I might be there for a while. I could only wait and see at that point. I told my mom that I was going to close my eyes until the nurse came in for my X-ray, so I could at least rest for a few minutes before the bad news began.

CHAPTER 10: DIGGING DEEP

My rest was short-lived as a nurse came in and told me it was time to get my X-rays. As I got in the wheelchair, she asked me what was going on and how I was doing. I kept the story short and said that I was doing okay.

In reality, I wasn't okay. I could barely breathe; how was I anywhere near okay? In part, I wanted to calm my own fears. I didn't want a pity party from anyone. I just wanted to get better and leave the hospital.

Interrupting my internal discussion, the nurse asked, "What happened to your knee?" I looked down and realized I was bleeding. In a state of confusion, I pulled my shorts back to see a small scrape with a trickle of blood coming from my knee. I told the nurse that the scrape must have happened when I fell at the track, but it was easily overlooked when breathing was my number one priority.

When we arrived at the X-ray room, I was told the doctor wanted to check for a broken rib or something of that nature, which could be causing my pain. I was skeptical, knowing I had not done anything which would cause a broken rib. But, I followed instructions.

I was told to lay flat on the table and put my arms above my head. It sounded simple enough, but as soon as I raised my arms, intense pain shot up my side. Instinctively, I dropped my arms. Each time I tried to comply, the pain became too severe. The technician told me that he would try to hurry if I could hold still for just a few seconds.

I took as deep of a breath as I could and quickly raised my arms above my head. I had to squint my eyes and clinch my fists in order to keep my arms up. I fought the pain with all I had, but I couldn't hold this very long. After 10 or 15 seconds, the operator told me that he got the pictures he needed.

I curled up in a ball. It's amazing what someone can do when they put their mind to it. In that moment, I couldn't let pain limit me. I had to think past it because there was clearly something wrong. These X-rays were key to understanding what was going on inside me.

I grimaced the entire ride back to my room. My sides were hurting so bad. I was struggling to breathe, and I was once again taking short, quick breaths. The nurse encouraged me to slow my breaths for fear of causing a panic attack. My body just wasn't giving me much choice. Breathing deep and slow caused too much pain. Keeping my breaths short didn't.

Back in the exam room, my mom had her eyes closed. She was exhausted considering it was after midnight. I wanted to rest just as much, so I also closed my eyes once we were alone.

The doctor woke us as he came in to discuss the results of my X-rays. He said there was good news and concerning news. I told him to provide the concerning news first.

He shuffled through his papers, pulled up the X-ray photos on a computer in the room, and motioned for my mother to come over to look at them with us. He began to explain that he had a good guess as to what was going on inside me, but the problem was that it could potentially be worse than a broken rib. The bright side, he said, was that I didn't have a broken rib. The doctor ordered light oxygen to support my breathing and a CT scan for in the morning to confirm his suspicions. I tried my best to remain positive.

A few minutes after the doctor left, a nurse took my mom and me to a regular hospital room. I felt bad that my mom had to sleep in a leather recliner near my bed, but she was never one to complain if she was taking care of loved ones.

Sleeping for me was near impossible. Any way that I laid, I was in pain. Finally, I dozed off and was able to rest for almost two hours.

I woke up to an essentially pitch-black room when I heard a knock on the door. A nurse walked in to check my vitals and ask me if everything was okay. I was very thirsty from breathing in the dry oxygen, so I asked for a cup of ice water.

I found a clock in the room which read 2:30 AM. The nurse came back into the room with a rather large jug of water that was refillable. When I asked if I could use the restroom, the nurse asked if I needed help. Being a 20-year-old guy, I declined.

I lumbered my way over to the restroom inside my room and did what I needed to do. As I opened the door to return to my bed, I could already feel myself getting winded. I had my oxygen off for less than five minutes, and I was already struggling to breathe. In that moment, I was petrified.

I returned to my bed and the oxygen as quickly as I could. I felt dependent on the oxygen already, and the thought of that terrified me. Images of myself pulling around an oxygen tank for the rest of my life flashed in my head. The unknown future scared me.

As I laid awake, unable to sleep, I could not shake those thoughts. I'd occasionally nod off for a few minutes, but the pain, frequency of nurses checking on me, and my fear kept me from resting for long.

Finally, the sun peaked into my room. A nurse and doctor came in to describe the battery of tests I would have that day, including the promised CT scan. Thoughts of the painful X-ray came flooding back. I knew I would have to dig deep to survive the day.

The nurse refilled my water and took my request for some orange sherbet and juice. Not exactly the breakfast of champions, but I wasn't hungry.

My dad came in and asked me how I was doing. I replied that I was tired and wanted to be home. Both parents chuckled as they tried to encourage me and be optimistic. I so badly wanted to share their optimism, but I had no clue what was wrong with me. The very act of breathing caused me pain, and we still had no diagnosis.

The three of us sat in my room for a while, and I eventually ate my sherbet. I tried to rest while waiting on someone to come get me for my CT scan. A short while later, a man wearing a long, white coat walked into my room and asked for my name and birthday. Once confirmed, he said, "I'm here to take you to get your CT scan."

I thought, "Here we go; this is it." The pessimist in me wanted to warn my parents of what could happen during the scan, while the budding optimist in me wanted to downplay the situation. I told myself, "It's okay. You've survived worse than this; you can survive this as well." I chose to just smile at my parents and tell them I'd be back, as I pushed down my fears.

Yet again, I was being wheeled down the long corridors of the hospital. My nervousness grew with every passing second. We passed through two secured doors before entering a large room with a long and circular machine in the center.

Picture a metallic bed with a large, metallic donut-shaped object encapsulating it. I took one glance at this machine, and I was already internally terrified. I knew that the pain that I was about to endure was inevitable. The only question was if I could handle it or not. The one thing I had going for me was that I had been through this pain once, so I believed I could do it again.

As I was positioned on the bed, I tried to take a deep breath to relax, but deep breaths just caused the pain in my sides to spike. I laid flat and informed the machine operators that I was going to keep my arms at my sides for as long as possible because it was going to cause me severe pain when I had to raise my arms. They seemed okay with this as they were still preparing the machine.

I was unable to shake the feeling of dread for what was coming. My heartbeat was slowly increasing. I just wanted this to be over. One of the assistants came over and told me that they'd have to remove my oxygen during the scan because it would interfere with the pictures. My heart raced faster. I was then told to raise my arms.

I slowly put my arms over my head. Pain instantly shot up my sides. I let out a groan and told the operator to go ahead and start the process because I wasn't going to be able to hold this very long.

The metallic table I was laying on started sliding through the donut-shaped hole. I was trying so hard to keep my arms where they were as the pain became more intense with each passing second. It felt as if this machine was moving at a turtle's pace. A bad chain reaction was stirring inside of me.

The pain was causing my heart rate to increase, which was causing my breathing to speed up. My rapid breathing was causing more pain and giving me anxiety. I couldn't hold my position for much longer. My energy was depleting and so was my will power.

I tried to judge how much longer I would have to hold my position. I was roughly 80% through the donut-shaped structure. Could I hold for the final 20%? I tried to convince myself that I had no other choice. I told myself that as soon as I cleared the donut, I was taking my arms back down by my side.

Finally, I cleared the donut and dropped my arms. I was struggling to breathe way more in that moment than I had been at any point since coming to the hospital the night before. I genuinely felt like I couldn't take in any oxygen. I motioned for someone to come over, so I could have access to the oxygen again. After what felt like an eternity, the assistant put my nosepiece back on. I tried to take in as much oxygen as I could, but the output of the oxygen was not enough. I asked if they could turn up the output but was told I had to have my doctor's approval to do so.

I tried my best to regroup as I was wheeled back to my room. I reported to the nurse pushing my wheelchair that I was having trouble breathing and that I was still in a considerable amount of pain. I don't know if it was the tone of my voice, my labored breathing, or the look of fear on my face, but the nurse quickened her pace. Once back in my room and on my bed, she checked my oxygen level again.

My oxygen had dropped to 60 percent. The look on the nurse's face as she reported my status over the phone startled me. I looked over at my parents who were equally as concerned as they overheard the nurse talking. My mom began to speak but was interrupted by the nurse who informed us I was being moved immediately to the Intensive Care Unit or "ICU." The announced move only served to punctuate what I already knew; something was seriously wrong.

I had reached deep into my soul to survive the pain of the CT scan. Little did I know how much deeper I would need to reach to survive what was to come.

CHAPTER 11: CALL TO ACTION

The nurse, having received permission to do so, increased the output on my oxygen tank and left to find assistance in moving me to the ICU. My parents asked me what had happened. Through labored breaths, I reported what had occurred during the scan. I began coughing as I struggled to breathe.

I was soon wheeled to the ICU. The doctor that ordered my CT scan walked into the room along with my parents soon after I got settled. He requested a second chair be brought in, so both my parents could sit down.

He then looked at my mom, dad, and I, and said, "While we are waiting on the chair, I'd like to discuss some things. Forest, obviously you're having a lot of trouble breathing. We are going to be doing a blood test on you soon to see if there is some kind of bacterial infection that is slowing your lungs' ability to intake oxygen. We have increased the level of your oxygen, so hopefully that at least alleviates some of your struggle for the time being." He then told us I would be in ICU for at least 48 hours.

For whatever reason, everything in the room began to fade out. I could hear the noise of the doctor saying something else to my parents. I could hear other background noises like the ping of my heart rate monitor, but it was as if I wasn't actually hearing anything. I began to zone out and become philosophical.

I thought back to my grandma's eulogy and the metaphor of the tree. In that moment, I knew that even I had taken the ability to breathe for granted. It was almost as if Life was trying to remind me of my lack of gratitude. How could something as precious as a breath ever be taken for granted? There are an infinite number of things that people benefit from in life that we never see, and we take them for granted. To be fair, people don't even appreciate what they can see the majority of the time, so how could one expect people to appreciate the things they can't see? Is that an unfair assessment, or is it simply true?

I finally snapped out of this train of thought when the doctor said my name. I blinked my eyes a few times, and I raised my eyebrows to acknowledge the doctor getting my attention. He then told me that he would return soon as the results for my CT scan came back. I nodded as if to give approval, and the doctor walked out of the room.

While waiting for the test results, I tried to catch up on rest that I didn't get the night before. I dozed in and out for a while until my ICU nurse came in. She said her name was Brenda and told me to call her by her first name. She seemed very caring from the moment she came in and introduced herself.

Brenda asked if there was anything I needed or if I was ready to order lunch. I told her that I wasn't hungry but that I just wanted some ice water and sleep. She abided exactly by what I asked for and said that she would leave me alone for an additional hour, so I could rest. She couldn't allow for any more than an extra hour though as ICU patients have to be monitored closely.

She brought back the water, and once she left, I fell asleep for an hour-and-a-half or so. It felt amazing to steal a bit of sleep because I basically hadn't rested in over a day. I was awakened by the sound of my parents talking. I gently opened my eyes to see my Grandma Pam and Grandpa Forest sitting in chairs talking to my parents. If you're wondering, I'm the third Forest in my family. Forest is my grandpa's name that was passed to my dad and then on to me.

My Grandma Pam waved at me and smiled, and I couldn't help but smile and wave back. My Grandpa Forest noticed me waving at my grandma and said, "Hey there, Big Bear! How are you?" Big Bear was always the nickname he gave me. I instantly smiled. I looked at him and jokingly said, "I've definitely been better." He chuckled and retorted with, "I bet you have, but we are all right here to fight with you."

I didn't show it in that moment, but you wouldn't believe how much those words meant to me. Having someone that you love telling you that they are there to fight right behind you is such an empowering feeling. People lose battles of this nature when they have to fight them alone. Having the support of people that care about you can definitely be enough to push you to victory. Once again, I realized that I had something to fight for. I had a reason to not give up because my family wasn't giving up on me, and I knew they never would.

A knock on the door caught all our attention. It was the doctor with my scan results. He walked over to a computer in the room and began entering some information.

He then opened a folder that he had brought with him and pulled out the pictures that had been taken in the CT scan. He said, "Forest, looking at your pictures makes it very easy to understand why you're having so much trouble breathing and the associated pain. If you look at the scan, do you see how this picture is primarily black, and only roughly 25 percent is white?" I nodded and asked what that meant.

He then pointed to the white section and explained, "This white section is the operating portion of your lungs, and the black on the bottom is essentially shut off. What this means is that you are essentially only able to access a quarter of your lungs at the moment."

I didn't know how to process that statement. I didn't have the chance to as he continued with, "Once I saw that your lungs were in this state, I looked back at your initial X-ray and was able to see that you have fluid on your lungs. This combination is usually a sign of progressed Pneumonia."

I was in shock. How did I get Pneumonia? What exactly did "progressed" mean? How was that possible?

Without me having to ask, the doctor said that he wasn't sure how

I could have gotten Pneumonia, but there was a high likelihood that's what I had. He then told everyone not to panic from the news. We may not have panicked, but we were certainly concerned.

The doctor then proceeded to tell me that I was going to be put on a machine called a CPAP, which stands for "Continuous Positive Airway Pressure." I asked what that was, and the doctor explained a CPAP machine forces large amounts of oxygen into your lungs and helps you breathe through an attached mask and tube.

It sounded kind of intimidating from the description. I proceeded to ask, "So, what exactly is the purpose of the CPAP machine other than to help me breathe?"

The doctor paused briefly and said, "I'm going to be honest with you, Forest. The CPAP machine is usually an escalated measure that is necessary when breathing becomes very difficult. Don't be afraid when I say that it's usually an emergency measure. It usually helps people in your condition quite a bit."

All I could think of was the idea that the CPAP machine sounded like a "last resort." I hoped it wasn't, but at that point, I was so used to bad news that it probably should have concerned me even more than it did.

I couldn't help but feel a little mentally defeated in that moment. I mean, I had weathered an emotional storm in the form of losing my grandma and being cheated on, and I had already been through severe pain with kidney stones. Was this going to be the end of my story? Had I survived everything else just to come up short now? What had I done to deserve that kind of punishment?

The doctor stood up and told us that someone would be coming in very shortly to administer the CPAP as he wanted to get me breathing properly as fast as possible. I nodded, and he walked out of the room.

I wanted to cry so bad. I wanted to break down because I had genuinely had enough at that point. I was never one to victimize myself or wallow in self-pity, but I felt like Life was just kicking me while I was down. I knew I didn't deserve all that was happening to me. I had the mental wherewithal to overcome what I had been faced with before, but this almost felt cruel.

I didn't want to cry in front of my family, though. I had to show them that I believed in survival and that I wasn't going to give up. Like I said, I knew they weren't going to give up on me, so I had to return the favor. With the prior events, I was fighting for myself, but in that specific moment, I was fighting for them. This was going to be my most difficult challenge yet.

Within a matter of a few minutes, two ladies came in to set up the CPAP machine. The mask I was given was so large and obtrusive that I could hardly see around it. One of the women explained, "This machine will give us a constant reading of your oxygen levels. If the machine starts beeping faster, your oxygen levels are decreasing. Right now, you're in the mid- 80's, and we are looking to get you into the 90's with the CPAP."

When the machine was set up, I was told, "When I hit this button, you're going to have a large amount of air pumped into you. It is normal to be startled at first, so don't get panicked; that will only make things worse."

When the machine was turned on, it genuinely felt like someone took my lungs and squeezed them like an empty two-liter bottle. It didn't hurt necessarily, but it wasn't comfortable either. Another pump came through, and I could already feel my heart rate beginning to rise. I had to synchronize my breathing to the machine, and it was starting to give me anxiety. After another pump, I heard the oxygen machine start to beep a bit faster, and I briefly glanced at the reading. It read 79. My oxygen was decreasing. How could this be?

Another pump and more anxiety came rushing at me. My heart monitor was starting to beep now as well. The oxygen reading was at 71. I could hear my mom and dad beginning to ask why my oxygen was falling, and my heart rate was rising. Another pump. I was completely out of sync with the machine now, and it essentially was breathing for me.

The nurse was encouraging me to synchronize my breathing with the machine and to relax. How could I do that? This machine was forcing air into me before I had the opportunity to rest in between breaths! Another pump. My oxygen machine was beeping like crazy. The reading was 61... 58... 55. More pumps kept coming, and I felt that I was beginning to fade. This was it, I thought. This might be the end of my story. I might die right here in front of my family. It seemed dramatic, but it wasn't. It was the realest thing I've ever felt.

Everything was fading to darkness, and my will to keep going was disappearing into the shadows. I was officially losing hope. I'd been through so much recently. I'd been through heartache and pain, but I thought this was what was going to be the nail in my coffin. I believed this almost entirely until I heard the most motivating few words that I have ever heard in my entire life. I heard my call to action.

My mom was clearly becoming upset. Through my panic and my fear and my waning hope, I overheard one sentence that would forever change my life. One of the machine operators said, "Mrs. Runnels, if the CPAP doesn't help your son, we really don't know what will."

My mother was being told I may not make it. Immediately, a fire lit inside of me. In that very moment, I made the decision to fight.

In that moment, I gained a new resolve. Never again, would I EVER let something take my hope away. Never again, would I EVER let something keep me down or feel defeated. Never again, would I EVER settle for anything but prosperity and positivity.

And NEVER AGAIN, would I EVER think that my life wasn't worth fighting for. I was going to beat this. I was going to put Pneumonia on my list of things I'd defeated just like all the other things that tried to hold me down. This was *not* going to be the end of my story.

CHAPTER 12: FATHERLY ADVICE

The CPAP machine had put me in a state of feeling completely zoned out. It was as if the outside world was drowned out, but I was focused on synchronizing with this machine, so it could do what it was supposed to do.

I felt a touch on my left arm that broke the trance-like state I was in. I opened my eyes to see my dad looking at me. Once he saw that I was responsive to his presence, he gave me *that* look. When I refer to "that look," I mean it was the look that he always gave my sister and I when he was serious about something. Normally, it was a look that was given to us when we were in trouble. I knew I was obviously not in trouble in the regard of doing something wrong in this case, but I knew what the look meant.

He said to me, "Listen. I know this is tough. As a parent, it's hard to see your kid struggling with any facet of life, but I need to tell you that you have to focus and breathe here. There is no other choice but to succeed. I know it's not easy; believe me, I get it. You have to focus and breathe."

He was right without question. There are reasons, and there are excuses for things in life. I had a reason to be struggling to breathe, but there was no excuse for not focusing and trying harder to pull that air in and let it go in tandem with the artificial help I was receiving. Now that I had my epiphany moment, and my dad was giving me a pep talk, I was ready to focus my entire mindset on overcoming this illness.

I was able to somewhat synchronize with the machine a bit, and my heart monitor was starting to beep slower gradually. The oxygen, despite dipping as low as 50, slowly started to rise, as well. It was rising a few points at a time until it got back to the high 80's! It never quite reached 90, but it was still progress. I did feel as though the CPAP machine had opened my lungs a bit. It wasn't necessarily the way that I would have liked my lungs to heal, but it was what had to be done.

All my vitals were stabilizing, and I could tell that everyone in the room was shocked. No one was expecting me to recover the way I did- especially not as fast as I did. While my oxygen was plummeting, I could tell that the levels of hope in the room were falling. But a miracle happened, and I survived.

For just a moment, I looked up to the ceiling. I wasn't looking at the ceiling; I was looking through it. I knew that my grandma had helped me recover. It was as if Life was trying to teach me a lesson about appreciating what I did have, and my grandma had stepped in to defend me because she knew that I understood the message.

The room was completely silent except for the lady machine operator taking off my mask. I believe everyone was trying to process what they had just witnessed. To be fair, I hadn't processed what had just happened either. I mean, I was essentially halfway dead and made almost an immediate improvement. That would take anyone a few moments to process.

The two operators gathered all their equipment and wheeled the CPAP machine out of the room, so it was just my family and I again. A few moments passed, and my Grandpa Forest broke the silence by asking if I felt that the machine had helped. I told him, "To be honest, I kind of have mixed feelings about it."

I paused as I tried to think of how to explain what had happened to me. I then continued, "I overheard the lady telling my mom they didn't know what else to do if the CPAP machine didn't help. It made me realize that I had to fight to overcome this. I knew I couldn't just lay there and hope; I had to focus on the task at hand and complete it. Once I shifted my mindset to fighting this illness, that's when I started breathing the way I was supposed to. I'm not really sure if it actually helped physically or not, but it helped mentally without question."

I saw my mom getting emotional as she wiped away a tear. I asked, "What's wrong, mom?"

"I thought I was losing my baby," she said sobbing. I looked at her with a small grin and said, "I told you I wasn't gonna let you miss me, and I meant it." She grinned from the joy of me keeping my promise to her.

For the remainder of the day, I had little appetite. I tried to rest as it had been over 36 hours with almost no sleep, but it was difficult. Not only were nurses coming into my room every 45 minutes; I was also now going to be having breathing treatments every three hours, which was something I found annoying and uncomfortable from the beginning.

At the end of the day, my Grandma Pam and Grandpa Forest got ready to leave. For several years, my grandma had been in a wheelchair as Parkinson's Disease robbed her of her mobility. This never kept her from seeing her grandkids as often as she could. As my grandpa wheeled her towards the door, I saw grandma motion for him to bring her over to my bedside.

When she was close enough, she grabbed my hand and told me "You're going to be okay. Mamaw won't let anything happen to you." She then smiled at me with a soft, warm expression on her face that was reflective of her soul.

The emotion I felt can't really be described. It was a sense of security that made me feel protected. It was very comforting.

As my grandparents left, all I could think was how blessed I felt. I couldn't have asked for a better family. They have always been such remarkable and supportive people in my life, and I can never thank them enough for all that they've done.

My dad prepared to leave to get dinner for himself and my sister. He told me that he'd be staying with me the following night, so my mom could get a night of sleep in a real bed. I looked forward to it, and he felt the same.

My dad and I always had a lot in common. In fact, we practically have the same mind. We think the same, say the same things, and have almost identical outlooks on life. That's why it was always so easy for me to connect with my dad. Don't get me wrong, I connect well with both my parents, but my dad and I are almost always on the same page in essentially any discussion.

I'm proud to say that I'm a lot like my dad. You really won't find a better guy. He's the hardest working man I know. He is unselfish, loyal, and such a great leader. Never once has my dad ever led me down the wrong path. Sure, he's made his share of mistakes; we all have, but I knew he always had his kids' best interest at heart.

When I was very young, my dad used to always sing "Just the Two of Us" by Will Smith to me. That song is such a great representation of my dad's love for both of his kids. There are lessons in that song that I could point to that perfectly describe how he parented us, but there are two in particular that I will always remember. The first is that there is no shame in crying. The second is to let God handle disrespect from other people because having hatred in your own heart will consume you.

Think about the meaning in those words. Usually, men are taught to not show any signs of weakness, but my father didn't raise me to bottle emotions up and feel nothing. He raised me to put everything I have into what I love. Sometimes, when you care about others or things that are important to you, you cry, and that's okay.

My dad always taught me to be the bigger person, regardless of how others treated me. He taught me to defend myself under the right circumstances. However, he emphasized integrity and taught me to never stoop down to someone else's level. I learned that the person extending an olive branch to someone else is always the happiest of the two. My dad taught me to fight hatred with kindness and love.

After my dad headed home, I was determined to fall asleep because I was completely exhausted. It had been a long couple of days, and my mind was as fatigued as my body. When a nurse came in to check on me, I requested some uninterrupted privacy. I needed to rest. She compromised by agreeing to check on me every 45 minutes while delaying breathing treatments until the morning.

After sleeping for six or seven hours, I woke up finally feeling rested, which was refreshing. I began my morning with a breathing treatment and a visit from my lung doctor. The doctor gave me some exercises to do to strengthen my lungs. I worked hard at this for several hours off and on. My goal was to minimize any pain I might experience when my next X-ray was ordered. I did not want to go through the previous kind of pain again.

My dad came back to the hospital late that evening, and he brought my sister with him. They brought dinner with them, so they could eat with my mom. My dad had offered to buy me food, but I declined. I was still not hungry for some reason. I had only eaten one cup of sherbet since I'd been in the hospital, which is obviously not a lot considering I'd been there almost two full days now.

At around 8:00, my mom asked my sister if she was ready to go home, so she could take a shower and get some sleep. They both gathered their things and came to give me a hug before leaving, both telling me they loved me.

When they left, it was just my dad and me, and we turned on ESPN. The Oklahoma City Thunder and Golden State Warriors were scheduled to play in the NBA playoffs. The game didn't start for a few minutes, but we figured we would watch the pregame show.

Almost on queue, a knock at the door was followed by, "Hi, I'm Robert from Respiratory, and I'm here for your breathing treatment." My dad and I looked at each other and couldn't help but laugh. The manner in which the clinicians from Respiratory announced themselves had become a joke with my family.

I did the breathing treatment, but afterwards I asked Robert from Respiratory if I could once again delay treatments until the morning. He told me that I had the option to completely decline the breathing treatments if I didn't want them as I was old enough to accept or decline treatment. I made a mental note of this for future reference and thanked him as he left.

"Well that was a relief, huh?" my dad said.

"Yeah, no kidding. If I had known that I was able to decline those, I would have turned them down several times." We both were chuckling, when I said, "Dad, do you think I'm gonna be okay? Like I mean more than just health-wise. Am I going to recover from all of these bumps in the road?"

Without hesitation, he said, "I have absolutely no doubt that you will be." My dad then gave me some of his best advice.

"If that's the case, then you can only survive going forward. The road of life is full of bumps. But, there is always a correct path to take. You will run into things that slow you down or make you go a different way; just don't ever turn around. Keep going forward until you reach your destination. You're a strong kid, and I know you have a fighting spirit in you. I raised you and your sister to never give up.

"There will be times where you'll want to quit because quitting seems easier than fighting, but do you think that anyone who was ever great gave up? No, they never gave up no matter how many times they failed. Michael Jordan didn't make his varsity basketball team at one point. He never gave up, and he ended his career as the greatest of all time. Tom Brady was drafted in the 6th round of the NFL draft, and now he is the greatest ever. Eminem lived in his mom's trailer for who knows how long, but he kept writing his songs until he became the greatest lyricist of all time.

"Life will get rough, but I'll always be here to guide you, and I'll never let you fall, son. Just don't ever forget that I always have your back."

CHAPTER 13: THE ROAD HOME

My dad and I watched the game that night and then fell asleep. Surprisingly, I got a decent night of sleep that night, interrupted only periodically by nurses doing their job.

In fact, it was about 8:00 AM the following morning when a knock on the door was followed by, "Hi, I'm Daniel from Respiratory. I'm here for your breathing treatment." I wasn't as annoyed this time since they honored my request to let me have a night without a treatment. Mid-way through the treatment, my lung doctor walked in with my nurse, and they were both entering some information into the computer in the room.

My doctor looked at me and somewhat cheerfully said, "Forest, I have some pretty good news. It looks like you're going to be able to leave ICU here in just a bit. Your numbers are stabilizing enough that you can move to a more private room that doesn't require the nurses to come in every forty-five minutes like they're made to up here. It should be easier for you to get some rest down there, and hopefully you can begin your process of heading home. We are shooting for sending you home in two days, which means you'd be hopefully going home sometime Friday."

Wow, what a relief! That was the best news I'd had in a while! I gave the doctor a thumbs up since I couldn't quite respond to him verbally with the breathing treatment in my mouth. My dad grinned at me and mouthed, "I told you you'd be okay."

I believed that I would be as well, but it was just nice to have reassurance. The doctor left the room, and my dad gave my mom a call to tell her the good news. Once the call ended, my dad told me that she was already on her way to come back to the hospital to see me, which was nice to hear. I was so happy to know that I was on the road to recovering and going home that I was just ready to get the next couple days over with. I was so ready to return home and hopefully put an official end to my run of bad luck.

After twenty minutes or so, my mom walked into my room with a big smile on her face. Before we got a chance to speak, a pair of nurses came in to move my bed down to the new room. My parents told me that they'd meet me down in the new room, but they were going to get breakfast together in the cafeteria first.

The nurses rolled my bed and all other necessary medical equipment down to the new room. It was quite the upgrade from ICU. I had my own full bathroom. My ICU room only had a pull-out toilet that was open to the rest of the room, and who can use the restroom in that circumstance? The room had an additional chair, and the best feature was that I had my own shower! I was beyond excited to be able to take a shower.

I hadn't fully bathed in almost three days, which is a long time for me. I typically shower every day, so I felt disgusting at that point. I couldn't wait to feel the water run down my body as the only form of cleansing I'd had since going to the hospital was a nurse helping to wash me off in the ICU. The thought of the warm water and soap running through my hair and down my body made me happier than it probably should have.

Without hesitation, I asked the nurse when I was able to use the shower, and she said that she would have to ask my doctor if it was okay that I could use the shower unattended. That made sense to me, but I told her that I felt comfortable to shower in there once my family returned to the room. She said that she would relay the message to my doctor and would get back with me as soon as she could.

I turned on the TV in my new room, and my phone vibrated. I checked the notification, and it was a text from Dexter that read, "Hey buddy. How are you doing in the hospital?"

I told him about the crazy events with the CPAP machine and that I had pneumonia. I also told him that I just moved to a new room. He then asked me what room it was because he planned on coming to see me that night. I had several friends who reached out to me saying they hoped I felt better soon, but Dexter was the only one who made an effort to come visit me. That meant a lot.

That's what friends are for. They're friends because they are there when no one else seems to be. Friends pick you up when everyone else knocks you down. This world would be a sad place without friends, and I'm grateful for all who have been there for me when things got tough.

My mom and dad returned from breakfast, and I informed them Dexter was coming later that evening. I also told them how eager I was to shower, and they both chuckled at my excitement. After all, it isn't every day that someone is ecstatic to step under a spray of hot or cold water, so I can understand how they found this to be humorous.

I was in such a good mood that I even ordered a full breakfast that morning. When the food arrived, I didn't eat all of it, but I did manage to eat for the first time since being at the hospital. Scrambled eggs, apple sauce, and toast never tasted so good, even if it was hospital food. It was a lot better than only drinking ice water.

The nurse returned and said, "I have talked to your doctor, and he has cleared you to take a shower if you'd like." With absolutely no hesitation, my reaction was an emphatic, "Yes!"

I asked for a towel and a new set of hospital robes to change into, and as soon as the nurse returned with those, I had her unhook all my machines, so I could make my way to the shower. The nurse showed me an emergency call lever in the shower that I could pull if I needed some assistance. I thanked her for her help, and I turned on the water.

There was a seat in the shower, so patients could rest if necessary. I sat on it and let the water pour down on me as I washed myself. Every second of it lived up to the hype I had built up in my mind.

I was probably in the shower for thirty minutes or so, but I was starting to feel tired. I'm not sure if it was just a lack of energy from laying in a bed for almost three days straight, or if it was from the heat of the water, but I heard my mom ask if I was okay.

I responded, "Yeah, I'm fine. I'm about to get out now."

I dried myself off and got dressed in the new set of clothes I was given, which also felt nice, but I was exhausted. I lumbered back over to my bed and sat down. I was also starting to feel nauseous, but I wasn't sure why. I don't know if it was the food I ate or the motion of moving after three days in bed. Either way, I was nauseous.

I rested my head on the bed pillow and tried to take a nap, but I couldn't get comfortable. All of a sudden, I covered my mouth and made a motion like I was going to get sick. I knew my mom would get the picture; she always did. She got up from her seat quickly and opened a cabinet in the room. She searched around for a moment and handed me a small bucket.

To spare the details, I did use the bucket, and my nausea subsided afterwards. I suppose that was my body making me pay for being in the shower for a half-hour, but oh well. The shower was worth it to me. Strangely, I had a newfound appreciation for showering. It's unbelievable what you can learn to appreciate when you're deprived of it even for a short period of time.

I laid around and tried to get some rest for the remainder of the afternoon, but I decided that I was going to try to start taking small walks around the hospital floor every so often just so that I could start to get some movement to my muscles and get my blood pumping. I knew that sitting still and lying in bed would only cause the fluid that was sitting on my lungs to remain there even longer. I was set on going home on Friday, so getting better was the only option.

On a similar note, I was ready to get back to the track. I strangely missed the place. You'd think I would be hesitant to go back up there considering what happened the last time, but that wasn't the case. I felt that going back up there and working my way to being healthy was the best choice for me. Plus, I was almost excited for the serenity that the track offered. Almost complete silence under the stars is a sure-fire way to clear your mind. Getting back to the track was now my goal. I wanted to be able to go home just so I could go back to the place that my mind was at ease. The place that my body and my mind would heal and strengthen; that is where I wanted to be.

I sat up in bed with a newfound motivation and waited for my nurse to come back in my room for a checkup. When she finally made her way in, I asked her if I would be able to take a small walk, so she helped me out of bed and got me a portable oxygen tank that I could walk around with. She walked beside me just in case anything went wrong, which was nice. The level of the hospital I was on was shaped like a large circle, and I made it all the way around back to my room without having to stop, which kind of surprised me.

I re-entered my room and saw Dexter talking to my mom and dad. My Grandma Pam, Grandpa Forest, and my sister were all in the room, as well. I was only gone roughly ten minutes, but apparently that was enough for several people to show up.

Dexter smiled at me and said "Hey buddy! How are you feeling?"

I chuckled. "Definitely been better, man. Thanks so much for coming!"

It was nice having so many people there that cared about me. I knew those people in that room would always have my back and support me through anything. The only person that was missing was my Grandpa Alvin. I wondered how he was doing, but I understood why he was unable to come to the hospital. He had been suffering from COPD for several years and had a weak immune system, so he was at risk being around sick people. I didn't want that for him, but I knew that he too would do anything for me that I ever needed.

Having those people with me showed me that I wasn't fighting alone, which was a nice feeling. I started to tear up, and my sister asked what was wrong.

I looked at everyone and said, "I just appreciate you all so much. You don't have to be here with me, but you are. I can't tell you enough how much that means to me." They all let out a collective, "You're welcome." I wanted to be sure they knew I appreciated their presence.

There isn't much more to speak of for the rest of the night as we all just talked and hung out in my hospital room until everyone headed home. I thanked everyone again for coming before they left for the night.

As Dexter was about to leave, he came over to give me a hug. He said, "Hey man, you have to get better, so we can go run some more. I leave for the Air Force in a month, and I've missed you up at the track this week."

I promised him I'd get better as fast as I could, so I could come up there even if I couldn't run right away. I told him I'd be up at the track my first night out of the hospital even if I had to bring an oxygen tank. He nodded as a sign of approval and left for the night.

Within an hour of everyone leaving, my mind was set on going to sleep and getting the following day over with as it was hopefully going to be my last full day in the hospital. I had a new resolve and goals already set. I was ready to go home.

CHAPTER 14: BREATHING FRESH AIR

I spent practically the whole next day trying to breathe as efficiently as I could and walking around the hospital level every hour or two to rehab myself. Only my dad and sister came to visit on that day, but it was fine. I didn't need the distraction.

In the evening, my nurse came in and said that they were going to try to let me go Friday afternoon. I couldn't have been happier! She said the only stipulation was that I would have to take a breathing test to see if I would need to be on oxygen when I went home. I was totally okay with that because I just wanted to leave. I was going stir-crazy sitting in the hospital, and I did feel considerably better than I did before I was admitted. I was still having minor pains from time to time, but it was only roughly 10% of what it was when I first entered the hospital several days before.

After another night sleeping in the hospital, I awoke in the morning totally excited with the hopes I'd be able to go home at some point that day. A nurse came in around 10:00 AM for my breathing test. Essentially, I had to breathe on my own to see what my oxygen level was without being supplied oxygen. If the level was below 90, I would have to be on oxygen while I was at home.

When I attempted the test, my reading was exactly at 90, which sounds great, but in reality, it was a bit misleading. It would be likely that once I went home, my oxygen level would fall without being supplied oxygen, which would probably put me right back in the hospital. I obviously didn't want that.

When the nurse saw this reading, she did me a huge favor. She told me that she and I were going to walk around the hospital without my oxygen on in hopes that my oxygen level would fall below 90, so that

I could have oxygen supplied to me when I went home. It sounded a bit scary, but it was totally worth it. To be honest, I kind of wanted the oxygen because I was afraid of what might happen without it.

We took a lap around the hospital, and my reading was an 88. Perfect. She recorded that my reading was an 88, which would qualify me to have oxygen. She put in the order right away and told me I was cleared to head home whenever the delivery arrived at the hospital.

That was easily the best news I'd had in quite a while. Several hours passed with me laying in the bed anxiously awaiting the arrival of my oxygen tank, which was delivered at 6:00 PM. A man wheeled the tank into my room and explained how to use it. I was getting a home unit, so I didn't have to lug around a tank while at home. I could just hook myself up to the unit and move about freely through the house.

A few moments later, the nurse came in with a wheelchair, and we started to make our way out to the lobby back on the first floor, and I got to see the front door of the hospital. I had to fill out some papers for being discharged, and then my mom wheeled me out to her car.

Wow … what a journey. The fresh air was invigorating after almost a week in the hospital. I slowly stood up from the wheelchair to get into my mom's car. She walked the wheelchair back to the hospital lobby, and we began our drive home.

I smiled the whole ride home with my newfound appreciation for life. I was never one to take things for granted, but I couldn't help but shake the feeling that I had taken life for granted. I was wrong for not seeing the beauty in life. I was wrong for not seeing the good with the bad. After all, without bad things happening, you can't fully appreciate the good things. You can't have good without evil.

After a half-hour drive, we arrived at home. My mom opened the garage door to park her car inside, and I could hear my dog howling when he saw us pulling into the driveway. He is a small dog. We were never really sure of his exact breed, but he definitely has some terrier in him. Either way, whenever he gets excited to see people, he always howls loudly. I opened the door inside of the garage, and the little guy came running up to me and jumped right on me. It was like he hadn't seen me in years.

Dogs are a blessing to the world. They love you unconditionally and miss you every second you're away from them. I was equally happy to see him, though. His name is Squirt. To be honest, I'm not sure why we named him that as a puppy, but it stuck instantly.

Even though I still didn't feel all that great, it was nice to be back home and away from the hospital. Before I forgot, I updated my boss at the gas station and let her know about my current situation. I told her that I was going to try to return to work in a week. She was very understanding and told me not to rush back.

I was a little apprehensive to return to my normal living routine, but I knew I had to get back out there. The world was going to keep spinning whether I was okay with it or not. All that I could think of was going back up to the track. I just wanted to sit in the bleachers and think for a while.

However, I decided to wait until the following night to go. I was pretty worn out and just wanted to sleep in my *real* bed. I decided to rinse off in the shower and hit the hay. When I opened the door to the shower, Squirt was laying on the ground right in front of the door waiting on me to get out. It was like he was afraid that I was going to stay in there and be away from him again.

I looked at the little guy and asked, "You want to go night-night?" Trust me, he understood what I meant. He followed me into my room and slept at the end of my bed that night.

The following evening, I told my mom and dad that I was going up to the track, but I told them not to worry as I wasn't going to be running with my oxygen tank. They laughed and just told me to be careful. I made the short drive there and decided to sit in the bleachers of the baseball field, which is in the same parking lot as the track. I figured the baseball field bleachers were smaller and would require me to walk up less stairs, which was much more appealing while lugging around an oxygen tank.

I walked up the ten or so steps to the top, and I was already out of breath. I knew the road to getting back into shape was going to be a long one if walking up ten steps already had me gassed. I sat down in the corner of the bleachers at the very top and leaned my back up against the fence that outlined the area. I closed my eyes and took a deep breath of fresh summer night air. I was capable of taking a deep breath for the first time in a week. My lungs couldn't quite handle breathing as deeply as they normally could, but I was able to breathe without pain, and that meant more to me than lung capacity at that moment.

Even though it sounds funny, I began to talk to myself.

"Wow … I have been through the ringer. I lost someone very important to me, I lost a relationship of more than six years, I endured kidney stones, and I wasn't far from dying in the hospital due to pneumonia… but I'm still breathing. I went through all of that in a three-month span, and I'm still alive. I wanted to give up numerous times. I wanted to lay on the ground and let life run me over, but I didn't. I chose to fight in all these situations. I chose to live."

There was a sense of pride that came over me as I sat there. I was proud to say that I made it through all of it. It gave me the feeling of being an underdog. I was counted out. I felt I wasn't supposed to make it out. Life didn't want me to come out of this situation. It was testing me to see what I was made of, and even though it wasn't easy, I passed the test. I couldn't help but grin at the thought of that. I wasn't supposed to be where I was, but yet I was there.

I'll admit, being sick in the hospital didn't take away the feeling of being depressed. To be truthful, it just distracted me from the feeling, but I can say in good faith that I learned a lot in the hospital. As people, we learn the most from tough situations. Pain is the greatest teacher. Nothing will teach you more than pain and suffering. It shows you that things can always be worse, so you should appreciate the good times more than you previously did.

I knew that I was still going to feel down for the time going forward because I had been through such a tough time, but I knew that I was on the way up now. Being on that CPAP machine and watching my life flash before my eyes was my personal rock bottom. It was a moment that forever changed my view of life because I knew what it was like to have the most precious thing that you're ever given almost taken away.

Is life a blessing or a curse? That's a question many people ask. Depending on your outlook, it can be either one. If you're more of a pessimist, you probably believe life is a curse. You might feel that you're ultimately born just to get a glimpse of the beauty of life only to eventually die. Personally, that's not my outlook. Prior to early 2016, I'll admit I was more of a pessimist in that I always assumed the worst was going to happen.

After the events of that fateful summer, my mindset shifted to being more appreciative of everything around me, telling myself that life is a blessing. All life is precious. From the fish swimming in the pond, to the birds flying in the sky, to human beings, all of it is beautiful and should be cherished to no end.

I never would have realized how amazing our world was if I hadn't gone through what I went through. I was going to see meaning in everything I looked at. I declared to myself that from that day forward, I was never going to take life for granted ever again. I'd never let a moment go by again that I lost sight of how blessed I am to simply be alive.

I sat up at the track until midnight that night. I was sending my mom text messages to let her know where I was and that I was okay just so she didn't worry. I figured that it was only right to keep her updated considering what happened the last time I was at the track.

Before I made the walk back to my car, I sent Dexter a text saying that I got to come home from the hospital and that I was planning on being back to running within a week. I had every intention of being at the track several times before then just to take in the night sky and think, but I knew that I obviously wasn't going to be able to do any physical exercise for the foreseeable future considering I had an oxygen tank. Either way, I was going to be back on the track running as fast as I possibly could. I missed the feeling of the night air hitting me in the face as I made my laps around. To be honest, I missed the feeling of exercising and feeling like I was burning up the calories and negative energy. I had to get back out there.

CHAPTER 15: BACK TO THE TRACK

The following week was good for me. I spent most of it resting and going up to the track at night just to clear my mind. Even if I didn't necessarily feel down, I liked just sitting in the darkness because it brought peace to my mind.

I had a check-up appointment with my lung doctor at the end of the week to see if I was able to be cleared to go back to work. Believe it or not, I was also permitted to be off of the oxygen tank as well as go back to work! It was truly awesome news that I wouldn't have to drag around a large oxygen tank anymore. I was very happy that I didn't have to return to college the following fall carrying around an oxygen tank. After all, I wouldn't have felt very "cool" walking around campus as a twenty-year-old with an oxygen tank, so that was a total relief.

I also texted my boss at the gas station to let her know that I could return to work whenever she needed me to since I was well enough to come back. She scheduled me to work that weekend but just for a short, four-hour shift so that I didn't have to do too much.

To be honest, I felt almost exponentially better than I did a week before, so I didn't think that working was going to be too tough. I assumed that I would probably need to sit down from time to time instead of standing for the whole shift behind the register, but I was sure that wouldn't be an issue.

I also told myself that I was going to begin trying to run again the evening after I worked. I figured this would give me a few more days to rest before I resumed my normal exercise and work routine.

I allotted myself a proper amount of rest before I went back to work, and I completed my first shift back at the gas station with no problems at all. I had several regular customers asking where I had been, and when they asked, I told them the short synopsis of what had happened. It was nice to know that people were thinking about me that didn't even really know me all that well outside of my workplace, but I suppose that is one positive of growing up in a small town.

Specifically, there was one customer who told me they knew I was in the hospital, but they didn't realize how serious my condition was. I confessed to them that I also was unaware of how severely sick I was until my lungs decided to give me a rude wake-up call.

I went home after my shift and told my mom and dad that it went well. I also told them that I planned on going for a run that night. They were a bit skeptical, but I told them that I was going to be asking Dexter if he wanted to go up with me so that I'd have someone there in case anything bad happened.

Knowing Dexter would be there made them a little less skeptical, so I went ahead and sent Dexter a text asking if he wanted to start running again since I was feeling better. He agreed to meet me at the track that night around 10:00.

The running went well. I couldn't quite go at my normal pace since my lungs were still recovering, and I had to stop and rest a few times, but overall, it went well. After we ran, Dexter and I sat at a picnic table close to the concession stand and talked about how crazy this year had been. We were at the track until around 1:00 AM just talking about life.

I asked him if he was ready to go to the Air Force, which at that point was only three weeks away. He explained that he was excited to go, but he knew he was going to miss his family and friends back at home. I knew that we all would miss him as well, and even though I had another person that was important to me heading off on a different path, I was happy for him. I knew that our friendship was like a brotherhood, and it wouldn't dissipate no matter how far away we were.

We both agreed to meet up at the track every night until he left for the Air Force. So, every night for the following three weeks, he and I went up to the track to run for a bit and talk about random things. Many times, he would leave the track, and I would stay behind for a bit afterwards just to be under the stars alone for a while. It was nice having someone to spend time with. There were also plenty of nights over the course of those three weeks that we would go on drives to random places such as a nearby Waffle House or Wal-Mart that were open 24/7 just to have something to do aside from running.

It was a lot of fun, and it helped relieve the feeling of being alone. There were clearly people that cared about me and wanted to be there for me. It can be hard to see that sometimes when you're depressed. A few nights before Dexter was supposed to leave for the Air Force, he told me that he was going to be having a going-away party for his friends and family. The party was to be on July 11th, the night before he would leave…

Without question, I was planning on going. He also invited my family to stop by because he had grown close to my parents and sister since we had spent so much time together. It was just going to be a small get together at his grandparents' house and a bonfire later at his house, which was right around the corner.

Those last few days passed quickly. When I arrived at the party, about 20 people were mingling and eating. I grabbed a plate of food and joined in on the conversation with the other party guests. After about 90 minutes, the party migrated to Dexter's house. His dad had left a few minutes before all of us to start a bonfire in their backyard. He left a crockpot of buffalo chicken dip to cook in the kitchen, which is one of the greatest things to ever be created.

The smell of the fire combined with the buffalo dip made for an incredible aroma that perfectly accentuated the mood of the evening. Dexter would be missed, but we all had this one last night together.

Once the night sky got a bit darker, we all began playing an old-fashioned game of "Truth or Dare." One of our friends, Austin, dared Dexter's brother Ryan and I to go into an abandoned house that shares a backyard with Dexter's house. As I didn't want to back down from a challenge, I accepted the dare. Ryan and I crept up to the house and looked for a way in. After fifteen minutes of looking for an entryway into the house, we thought to check the back door. To our surprise, it swung right open at the turn of the doorknob. Ryan and I looked at each other kind of surprised, but we entered the dark house.

There was a cloud of stagnant dust hanging throughout the three-story building. We were using our cell phones as flashlights to be able to navigate through the house. Technically, we only had to go into the house to complete the dare, so we had already completed our "challenge." But, we figured that we would go ahead and look through the house.

The first and third floors were empty except for some furniture, an empty beer can and a camcorder that had to be at least 10 years old. We didn't turn on the camera, for fear of what might have been recorded in the now abandoned house.

Easily the creepiest scene in the abandoned house came as soon as we walked past what appeared to be a young girl's room on the second floor. A wooden pony sat still in the center of the room, surrounded by clothing and toys. I looked at Ryan and said, "If that horse moves, I'm out of here." We both chuckled, but I totally meant it. On the third floor, Ryan and I decided to open the window and call out to the people sitting around the fire to let them know that we had made it all the way to the top.

When we rejoined the others around the bonfire, several people were surprised that we actually accepted the dare and admitted that they would not have gone into the house. I'll admit that I was a bit hesitant at first, but it wasn't all that scary once Ryan and I were inside.

Not too long after, my dad pulled into Dexter's driveway and joined all of us in the backyard near the fire. Before he had a chance to greet everyone, police sirens went off nearby, and we heard what sounded like a vehicle engine firing up aggressively.

A loud "BANG!" echoed from right in front of Dexter's house and a truck passed by going way over the speed limit. Curious, everyone hurried to the front of the house to check out what just happened and looked for what caused the loud noise. Once we reached the street, it became very apparent.

The street that Dexter lived on was small and narrow and was split in half by a public park that only had a small playground and a couple of benches. Tire tracks tore through the small park, and one of Dexter's neighbors had their fence completely demolished by the truck that came barreling through. The driver apparently was coming down the other half of Dexter's street and didn't realize the road was divided by the small park, so they drove straight through it.

Police pulled up in front of Dexter's house soon after and were asking us what we had seen and made sure that everyone was okay. Thankfully, everyone was just fine. The only thing that was really destroyed was the neighbor's fence.

After that excitement, I said my goodbyes to everyone. I was scheduled to open the gas station the following morning. I pulled Dexter aside and thanked him for being such a good friend to me when I needed someone. He said, "Of course, buddy. I know you'd do the same for me. That's what friends are for. I'll be in touch as soon as I get the access to use my phone." Since he was going to basic training, he wouldn't have access to his cellphone until September.

It was a bittersweet moment as I knew I'd miss having someone to go to the track with, but I was happy Dexter was doing something to better his life and that he was excited about it. I really wanted to head up to the track that night, but I decided against it since I had to be at work at 6:30 the next morning.

I made the short trip home and tried to rest. It was hard to fall asleep as I was thinking about how I'd be alone at the track every night again. As sad as this was, it didn't deter me from wanting to go. I had a purpose and a goal that I still needed to attain at the track, and that was healing myself both physically and mentally.

I was still far from where I wanted to be, but I knew that ultimately, I had to be the one that healed myself. I had to rely on myself to fix the issues I had inside of me. I knew I had people that cared about me. I knew those same people would do anything to help me get better as best they could. But only I am responsible for recovering and strengthening myself. No one was going to get better for me. I had made good progress towards fixing my mental health, but I still had plenty of distance to cover. My recovery was my responsibility.

CHAPTER 16: TAKING A CHANCE

I woke up the next morning and headed to work. I only had to be at work until 12:30, so I had plenty of the day remaining to do something afterwards. Aside from my typical job duties, I spent most my shift trying to look at Facebook's events page to see if there was anything that sounded fun going on once I got off work.

Nothing sounded super enticing, and most of the things that sounded intriguing were at least an hour away. I finally found an event at a nearby museum scheduled for the next day. It was an educational event celebrating the achievement of NASA sending a satellite to orbit Jupiter. The satellite was going to finally enter Jupiter's orbit, and it sounded interesting. Plus, it was a free event and open to the public.

That night, when I went to the track, I ran without my headphones on. I wanted the serenity of not hearing anything. As I sat in the bleachers afterwards, I felt incredibly lonely. I'm not sure if it was the lack of noise or the lack of another person's presence, but I felt completely isolated.

You would be surprised how much you learn about yourself when you are alone with your thoughts. You start to realize how you think without any influence. What goes on in your mind when other people aren't around to persuade you to think a certain way? Does the presence of another person help an overwhelmingly negative situation, or does it distract you from the real problem: yourself?

You are the bearer of all good and bad that comes your way. You can make any situation positive or negative if you choose. The outlook of any situation is completely dependent on your perception of it. Did something cause you pain? If so, it can be looked at simply as something painful, or it can be something that makes you stronger. Pain is the greatest teacher.

As I was sitting in the bleachers in silence that night, I chose to look at everything I had been through recently as an opportunity to learn and make my life better. Sulking in my own misery and waiting on things to turn my way was not going to be an option. If I wanted things to get better for myself, I was the one responsible for doing so.

Even though I had been shoved, knocked down, kicked while I was down, and spit on by life, I chose to look at my situation as a blessing. Think about it. My grandmother had passed away. I will forever miss her, but she is resting and is watching over me. Sure, I had been betrayed by Sofia, but I had an opportunity for a new relationship founded upon trust, long-term happiness, and commitment. I had been very ill, but I now had an appreciation for life and being able to breathe that I never would have had otherwise.

All these situations were challenges, but challenges should not be looked at in a negative light. Challenges are blessings and opportunities to learn. Even if you don't succeed with a challenge, that's perfectly fine. In any situation, you either win or you learn. You never lose until you give up.

I looked up to the sky and saw three lights flying in unison right above the track. The lights flew overhead to the West, and I gauged the speed to be rather fast. I'm not sure what caused these speeding lights, but it looked like three shooting stars flying together. In a way, it felt like the cosmos reminding me that I had so much left to see in this life. I had so much opportunity, and what I had faced was only a molehill compared to the mountain of life.

Although I had no idea what these lights were, I smiled as they flashed by out of appreciation for the blessings that I had. I looked straight into the sky and mouthed the words "Thank you." I then gathered my things and went home for the night.

I awoke the next morning and started getting ready for the NASA event, which started at noon. My mom walked into my room and asked where I was going.

"I'm going to a free event at Boonshoft Museum where they are doing a demonstration for the satellite that NASA sent to Jupiter. The satellite just entered Jupiter's orbit."

"Who are you going with?" my mom asked.

"No one. I was just going to go by myself," I replied.

She tilted her head and had somewhat of a sad expression on her face. She then said, "Well it's a Sunday, and your dad is off. We don't have anything to do, so we can join you if you'd like."

I grinned and said, "Sure. I'd love if you guys tagged along."

I could tell that my mom was offering to come just because she felt bad that I had no one to go with. Moms have an instinct for knowing when their children aren't happy. They also have a related instinct for trying to create happiness for their children in these same instances. From an optical standpoint, a twenty-year-old going to a free event at a children's museum alone on a Sunday afternoon probably did sound kind of sad.

My mom talked to my dad and told him where the three of us were going to go, and he was happy to join us. We all got dressed and had a quick lunch before getting into the car to head to the museum.

We left around 11:15. The drive to the museum was only about a half-hour, but my dad always liked to arrive early to places, so we left a few minutes earlier than we probably needed to. We pulled into the museum parking lot around 11:45 and made our way up to the front door. Even though there was a line of people in front of us, the auditorium could easily hold those gathered.

We made our way into the auditorium and got seated. The entire ceiling was a giant projector screen, which was impressive to look at. A man walked into the auditorium, and the lights dimmed. An image of Dayton's city skyline appeared on the ceiling. Normally, I wouldn't think of Dayton's city skyline as "majestic," but seeing it on this projector made it look beautiful.

More images of Dayton flashed on the screen that acted as an introduction to the presentation that would follow. A spotlight flashed onto the man up front, and he began to speak. The man welcomed everyone and explained what would be taking place during the rest of event.

The presentation itself was awesome! We saw stunning images of the satellite's travels. The aerial view of Earth, the deep reds of Mars, the mysterious void of outer space, and the massive planet Jupiter itself all made for astonishing views.

Seeing what life outside of Earth looks like is a very humbling experience. It reinforces the idea that our life here on Earth is so small, and since life on Earth is small, so are the problems that life throws at you. Any problem can be solved. Any mountain can be climbed; any body of water can be swam; any distance can be travelled.

The answers to your problems may not actually be in the stars, but you can always look to them for inspiration. On a clear night, you can see several hundred stars in the sky, and each one looks like a small white dot on a black canvas. In comparison to where you're at, they look very small. The ironic thing is that every star you can see in the clear night sky is so large that you can see it from millions or even billions of lightyears away.

Now picture your mind and your mental health as a clear night sky where the stars are the problems in your life. If you look at your problems from far away, they appear very small, but the closer you get to them the larger they become. Intuitively, your problems may also be larger than you give them credit for. You might try to compartmentalize your issues and act as if they are nothing to worry about, but in actuality, they're massive conflicts that need to be resolved. The stars can provide countless metaphors, but the metaphor of perspective is the greatest.

The presentation lasted roughly an hour and ended with the man thanking everyone for coming out. My parents seemed to enjoy the event, and I was happy I had people to share the experience with.

When we got back home, I told my parents that I felt like going to get ice cream, and I asked if they wanted me to bring them back some. They both declined but thanked me for the offer. I decided to go to my favorite ice cream place, Baskin Robbins. I have been to this Baskin Robbins so many times that I am considered a regular.

I pulled up to the drive thru window, and the manager greeted me with a friendly, "Hello!"

He recognized my car in the security camera, so he asked, "Would you like a small chocolate milkshake?"

"Yes sir; I would love that," was my response. We chatted for a moment as I paid for my order. The Dayton area has several metro parks. I drove to my favorite one which was a few minutes away.

The park is called Cox Arboretum. It has a butterfly house, several ponds that are full of life, flower gardens, several walking trails, and a large tower that gives a gorgeous view of the Miami Valley. When I arrived, I headed for the tower. Normally, I tend to be afraid of heights, but the view at the top was worth overcoming my fear.

At the top, I gazed around and saw the valley from an angle that is not accessible from many other places. Seeing the presentation at the museum inspired me to look at the world from a different perspective. Now, I understood that there was life below me. There was life everywhere, and life is beauty.

I returned home and relaxed the remainder of the afternoon, contemplating for most of the day on whether I wanted to go on a run that night or not. I ultimately decided I should. I needed to keep up the good habit of exercise for my physical and mental health, and I had a milkshake to work off.

As per usual, I drove up to the track once the sun set and started my typical routine of runs. It was abnormally warm that night, and I sat down on the track to rest for a moment. Once again, the lonely feeling consumed me. A moment of relaxation gave way to a moment of sadness. I desperately wanted someone to share my thoughts with. I wanted someone that I could tell all the amazing lessons that I learned over that summer. I wanted someone that I could take to get a milkshake at Baskin Robbins and walk with up the tower at Cox Arboretum to look at the valley below. I wanted someone that enjoyed looking at the stars on a clear night. I wanted someone that wanted to listen to me ramble on about some sort of philosophical topic for hours just because they wanted to know what was on my mind. I just wanted someone to share my life with.

My newfound appreciation for life made me want this more than I ever had before, but I had to start from scratch with someone. I had to make someone fall in love with me again. What if I found someone that I fell in love with, and it turned out just like my relationship with Sophia? What if I was rejected? What if girls mistook my genuine attempt at chivalry for a "sweet-talker" trying to take advantage of them?

What if I just wasn't as likable because my viewpoint on the world is abnormal, and I enjoy philosophy more than being "cool"? Should I even be thinking in this manner, or should I just put myself back out there?

I wasn't desperate to be loved or to be in a relationship. I just was desperate for some sort of companionship. I wanted someone to share my view of the world. A relationship or love would just be a bonus.

I finally decided to reach out and try to make new friends. In this day and age, that meant going to social media. Most things on Facebook never really interested me as I was never one to be vested in other people's personal lives. But, now, I decided to see if I could find someone to engage in conversation.

I liked the idea of a new experience, but the idea of sending a request to someone that I wasn't familiar with felt awkward. I closed the app for a few minutes and turned on the music on my phone. I wanted companionship, but I preferred it to be organic. I listened to the music for a few minutes and worked up the courage to open Facebook again.

I looked for people from college, knowing we would at least have something in common. I struggled to find people that I had been to school with as I only befriended a few in my first two years of college. That's when I scrolled across a picture of a girl with wavy blonde hair. She looked very familiar. I knew that I had seen her somewhere, but I couldn't quite pin where it was. Her name was Brittany.

We had one mutual friend, who a guy I had a previous class with. After a few minutes of thinking back, this girl reminded me of someone that was in my Freshman science class. She was beautiful, but I remembered her having darker hair, not blonde. I felt a bit like a stalker, but a quick look at her profile pictures confirmed she had darker hair the year before. Brittany had an unusual last name, which I remember the professor questioning how to pronounce. This had to be the same girl.

This is when the moment of truth came. Should I take the step and send her a friend request? Self-doubt crept into my mind. Before I could change my mind, I clicked the "add friend" button. There was no going back.

I looked up at the sky and decided that it was time to call it a night. I walked back to my car assuming my friend request would probably be deleted, and nothing would come of it, but at least I took a step at trying to move on. I could at least rest that night knowing I gave it an attempt. The worst thing that could happen is that nothing would change, and I would be in the same predicament the next day.

I laid in bed the entire night feeling weird for sending the friend request to Brittany. She probably didn't remember me since we hadn't had class for almost two full years. I finally convinced myself that it wasn't a big deal and went to sleep.

I woke up the next morning a little timid to check my phone to see if Brittany had accepted my request or not. There was no response yet, but it was only 7:00 A.M. It was likely that she wasn't awake yet. It was also possible that she could have just deleted the request.

"Meh, it's all good," I thought to myself as I sat up in bed. I convinced myself that I shouldn't get my hopes up because it was quite a long shot anyways. She was way out of my league, but it was worth a shot. At least I had taken the chance.

CHAPTER 17: A NEW BEGINNING

I walked to the kitchen to get some breakfast and told my mom good morning. I felt like telling my mom how lonely I felt, but no one wants to tell their mom about something like that. That's the epitome of pathetic, but I just wanted someone to talk to about it. I decided against mentioning my loneliness and opted to make typical small talk instead.

She asked what I had planned for the week, and I replied, "Work and running ... the only things I've done all summer." We both chuckled, but she had that sad look in her eye again. Moms can tell when their kids are hurting or when they need something.

I decided to go to a nearby park to shoot basketball until my shift later that night. I was shooting for a half-hour or so when my phone started ringing. I walked over to the table where I had placed my phone to check who was calling.

It was my mom. She just wanted to know if I was coming back for lunch, and I told her I was, but not for a half-hour or so. I hung up the phone and was about to resume shooting when a notification from Facebook popped up on my phone saying, "Brittany Wead has accepted your friend request."

I was extremely surprised! She must have remembered me, or she wouldn't have accepted my request! Now the question that I had to ask myself was whether or not I should initiate a conversation with her. My thinking was that since I sent her the friend request, I should be conservative about making another move. I didn't want to come across as too aggressive.

I was never the type of guy to assume that women naturally like me. In fact, I despised men who acted that way. Guys like that have always ruined the reputations of men that actually try to respect women. It was always quite the annoyance for me because my genuine attempt at chivalry has been mistaken as an attempt to "sweet talk" my way into "getting what I want."

I decided to wait before initiating any kind of conversation with Brittany. I didn't want to give off any sort of aggressive vibe. I resumed shooting basketball for a few minutes before heading home for lunch.

When I got home, Squirt greeted me at the door. It appeared my mom had given him a haircut since I left. Since his hair cut looked so cute, I decided to post a picture of us on my Facebook and Instagram accounts. As I sat down for lunch, I felt my phone vibrate a few times, but I didn't check it right away. When I did, there were probably fifteen notifications from Facebook and Instagram of people liking my photo. Much to my surprise, one of those people was Brittany! She liked my post on both Facebook and Instagram.

I wasn't sure what to do next. I spent time that night sitting in my usual spot at the track. I was excited about the thought of talking to Brittany and getting to know her, but my pessimistic brain kept asking me things like, "What if she doesn't like you? What if she finds you weird? What if she doesn't think you're good-looking? What if she actually has a boyfriend but just doesn't put that information online?" The very shy, optimistic portion of my brain only asked one question in return. "What if you don't give it a try?"

After a lot of back and forth, I decided that I was going to take a leap of faith and message Brittany in the morning. After breakfast, I walked into my mom's room where she was doing her hair.

"Everything okay?" She asked.

"Yeah …" I trailed off for a moment. It was awkward talking to my mother about this, but I needed some advice and encouragement.

"So, if you were me, and you knew this pretty girl that you met in college, and you just became friends with her on Facebook, and you wanted to get to know her, but you weren't 'available' when you knew her, would you try talking to her now, or would that be weird?"

"That's very specific," she said while chuckling. "I'm going to assume that all of that does apply to you?"

"It may, or it may not," I responded with my own chuckle.

She then said, "It's nice to see you smile. I haven't been blessed with seeing your smile very much recently. My advice to you is to give it a shot. Why not? What can it hurt to just say 'hi' to her?"

She had a point. There was no harm in saying "Hello."

My mom then continued by saying, "I promise you that one day someone will love and appreciate you the way you deserve. You can't be afraid to put yourself out there, and don't be afraid to give someone your all again just because you were hurt in the past. Treat every situation with a clean slate."

She was clearly right about that. I had to have confidence that I was good enough. I had to know that I was worth it.

A quick rush overcame me, and I sent Brittany a message on Facebook simply saying, "Hey! How have you been?" After what seemed like an eternity, a message popped up that read, "I'm good! How are you?"

She replied! I was so surprised that I didn't know how to comprehend it. I just knew that I clearly felt happy about it. We exchanged texts asking about school and how the summer went. With each message, my anxiety lessened. We ended up talking for almost an hour before she said she had to go to work and wouldn't be to use her phone. She ended the conversation temporarily saying, "I have to go, but can we continue this conversation after I get off work?"

"ABSOLUTELY!" I said as I was ecstatic that she wanted to talk to me again. Knowing that she wanted to keep the conversation going let me know that she at least found me interesting so far, and I was super excited about it. Just talking to Brittany for an hour made my loneliness dissipate significantly.

I had a reason to wear a smile on my face for the first time in months. I had spent months faking a smile to give the world the impression of being okay. I was smiling to everyone's face but crying whenever they left the room. But finally, my luck may have changed. I had reason for an actual smile. Something about talking to Brittany for an hour felt different. Obviously, I was coming off a long relationship that ended sourly, but something about talking to Brittany felt so natural and correct from the very beginning.

I had to get ready to go to work late that afternoon, so I put on my normal work attire and made my way up to the gas station. I was closing that night, but I was excited to know that Brittany would be texting me at some point. As I began to close the store just before 10:00, I got a text from Brittany saying, "Hey!!"

The grin on my face felt like it went from ear to ear. I got the cliché "butterflies" in my stomach just from this simple text message. It was such a happy feeling to feel like someone wanted to talk to me.

We sent text messages back and forth for about two hours that evening until she said that she was going to sleep because she was exhausted from her shift at work. I understood that completely, and I wished her goodnight. She told me that we could talk again the following morning if I would like, and my response was a heartfelt "Duh!!"

Even though I had worked for several hours, I wasn't tired yet, so I decided to go up to the track. For the first time in several months, I went up to the track without the intent to be sad. I went to the track to look up at the stars and say, "Thank you."

CHAPTER 18: HOLY

I didn't run that night; all I did was sit in the bleachers and stare up at the stars. I could tell that my luck was finally starting to shift. I learned something that night. I learned the meaning of patience.

Patience can be a hard skill to acquire, but it is very valuable to obtain. To some people, patience is simply waiting and hoping that something good happens. This gives the word a negative connotation. The people that view patience this way are wrong. Patience and perseverance go hand-in-hand. Patience means not expecting results to happen overnight. Patience means weathering the storm because you know the sun will shine once the rain ceases. Patience is never giving up and keeping your hope no matter how bleak the situation may be.

Patience isn't passive. You have to actively be patient. You have to be patient with those you love. You have to be patient with your goals and aspirations and realize that things take time to build. You have to choose to be patient and realize that some things take time and will power. Do you think that successful people just had a dream, and it came true the next morning? Well I have news for you. That's not how it works.

Learning the lesson of patience that night was one of the most important things I've ever learned. It changed my outlook on how I would approach tough situations for the rest of my life. I would no longer look at problems exclusively in the moment. I would look at problems as something that may take time to solve. Not every problem needs to be solved immediately.

I looked at the sky and said "Thank you" one last time before returning home and going to sleep for the night. It was the best night of sleep I'd had in months as I felt like I went to sleep stress-free. Learning an important life-lesson and having an awesome person to talk to made resting a lot easier.

Brittany and I talked every chance we got for the following several days. The only times we weren't texting was when she was at work, but we never ran out of things to talk about.

I found out that she has a dark sense of humor like me. Her birthday was only six days after mine. She is a Disney fanatic. We share very similar social views. Every message I received from her made me feel even more like this was a match made in Heaven.

After texting practically non-stop for about four days, Brittany asked me to hang out. I know what you're thinking. Why did I let her ask me out and not the other way around? For two reasons. One, my confidence was a bit damaged at the time, and even though I had no reason to be afraid, a small part of me was. Two, I have always been a man that believes that women should make the first move, so I don't ever feel like I'm making a girl uncomfortable. If a girl makes the first move, then she is clearly interested. Chivalry isn't dead; it's just dying, unfortunately.

My answer to Brittany's inquiry was obviously an emphatic, "Yes!" We discussed our schedules and decided to hang out Sunday, which was two days away. I offered to pick her up at her house and told her that I would plan the date.

She liked my plan, which meant I had a date to organize in my head. Luckily, I knew just where to take Brittany. A special occasion deserved a special outfit. I drove to the closest mall right away to look for an outfit, which is not normal for me. I hate shopping for clothes. I purchased a nice shirt and a pair of khaki shorts.

I arrived back home, and my mom knew something was up. "You bought clothes?" She asked in a very puzzled manner, but her confusion was understandable. I hadn't bought myself clothes in several years. Without much hesitation, she asked, "So when is your date with Brittany?" I smiled and told her it was Sunday evening.

She was very happy for me and wished me good luck. She told me that she knew it would go fine, but she wanted me to tell her about it afterwards. I told her I'd give her the details as long as it went well, and we both giggled.

Brittany and I both had to work the following day, but we talked whenever we had the opportunity. I decided to go to bed early instead of going up to the track like normal. I just wanted our date to come as soon as possible, so staying out late would just prolong the wait.

I awoke on Sunday, July 23rd. That was the day of my date with Brittany. After I ate lunch, I spent the majority of the afternoon getting ready. I showered, shaved, and made sure my outfit looked good. I put a lot of effort into my appearance for the date because I liked Brittany a lot already, so I wanted to impress her.

The drive to Brittany's house took about forty minutes, and my nerves were eating me alive the entire ride. I was equally excited and nervous to see her. I arrived at her house and parked my car on the street. As I knocked on her door, I heard what sounded like two dogs barking. Just a moment later, Brittany opened the door and greeted me with her beautiful smile.

She was wearing a lovely blue summer dress and asked me if I was ready to get going. I was so awestruck that I hesitated for a moment before saying, "Yes, absolutely."

We began walking to my car when she asked, "So, where are we going today?"

"It is a surprise." We both had already eaten so I asked if she liked ice cream. "Who doesn't like ice cream?" she retorted back with mild sarcasm. I knew just where to go.

The drive from Brittany's house to Baskin Robbins took roughly a half-hour. As I drove, we talked like we had known each other for years. Our chemistry was instantly amazing. She laughed at pretty much all my jokes (especially the dark-humored ones), and she made plenty of jokes herself. I already felt comfortable around her. I didn't feel the need to be superficial or act any certain way to impress her. I just had to be me.

Brittany had never had ice cream from Baskin Robbins before. She ordered a peanut butter cup milkshake, and I had my usual small chocolate version. She took a sip of hers, and her eyes got really wide. "Oh … wow, that's good," she said. I simply smiled and nodded. I then asked her if she had ever been to Cox Arboretum. She told me that she knew someone who had their senior pictures in high school done there, but she had never really seen the full park.

We made the short trip and walked around the park. We stopped from time to time to take in the beauty of nature. She really liked the pond with all the turtles as well as the small bridge that creates a path over the water.

Once we got past the bridge, I pointed out the large tower near the middle of the park and asked if she wanted to go to the top with me. She told me that she would love to, so we walked up the six-story tower and looked at the same view that I took in just a few days before.

A thought entered my mind. Earlier in the week, I so badly wanted someone to experience the beauty of the world with, and there I was. I stood at the top of a tower with a girl that minimized the beauty of the valley behind her. It was almost like the view without her was gray, but adding her to the scenery gave it color.

At that moment, it was like the final piece of my puzzle was finished. I already knew I wanted her to be the one that I witnessed the beauty of the world with. Something about her instantly stood out that made her different from every other person I'd ever met. It was always commonly said that when you find the one, you know it instantly. Brittany gave me that feeling.

I caught myself staring at her.

"Sorry, you just look so pretty," I told her.

She smiled at me while blushing and said, "Thank you."

I couldn't help it; she looked like an angel that had floated down from the sky and landed next to me. As much as I wanted to stay at the top of the tower and look out over the valley, I asked if she wanted to continue walking around the park.

We made our way down and followed one of the paths that went back into a wetlands preserve on the south side. The wetlands were ironically dry, so we walked around them and found a dried-up swamp area. She dared me to run out into the swamp, so I obviously had to do it. I jumped off the platform that we were on and ran into the barren land. The only thing I was afraid of was potential quicksand, but luckily there was none.

I ran back over to the platform and invited her to join me. "Come on down! The water is fine!"

Brittany chuckled and looked down at me. I offered my hand out to her, and she put her hand in mine allowing me to help her down. We walked out into the dried-up swamp together, and it felt like we were kids playing in the mud.

There was an innocence to the moment that felt beautiful. It was fun, and that was exactly what I wanted. We had only been on a date for an hour-and-a-half, but my soul felt restored.

We made our way back to my car, and I asked how long she wanted to stay out. She told me that it didn't matter to her, so I asked if she wanted to see my hometown. "Sure! I've had fun tonight so far." I was so happy to know that she was enjoying herself.

I warned her that my hometown was nothing special, but she did not seem to care. I drove by my house and pointed it out to her, I showed her the basketball court that I played at often, and lastly, I showed her the track that I had been going to every night. She already knew of my nightly runs, but I hadn't yet told her the reason why I had been running every night. I can only imagine she thought it was to exercise, and that was a part of it, but it wasn't the full story. My time to tell her the full story was still far away. I didn't want to lay on a depressing story to kill the mood. Plus, it was almost impossible to be upset or have dark thoughts while being with Brittany.

I had also told her my passion for looking at stars. It was a perfectly clear night, so I asked her if she wanted to sit in the bleachers and look at the stars with me. "I would love to," were the words she said.

We walked up the bleachers and sat down on the top row of seats. She sat next to me and laid her head on my shoulder.

"You're so different from every guy I've ever been with. Just the way you look at the world is so different. Most guys would have already made some sort of sexual advance at me by now, but you seem like you genuinely just want to spend time with me."

It was like music to my ears. That's the exact impression I wanted her to have. I didn't want to come off as a guy that only has one thing on his mind because I sincerely just wanted to love someone, and I wanted someone to love me in return.

You can't find true love if you're looking for someone who wants to immediately make a relationship physical. The best partners fall in love with you as a person before they fall in love with your body. Sure, there may be physical attraction right away, but if you want a successful relationship, your sole focus should be on falling in love with what is inside the person as opposed to how they look on the outside. Everyone has a physical appearance that will eventually wane and deteriorate, but the person on the inside will always be the same.

I thanked Brittany for her comment and replied: "I don't think you could understand how much that means to me. That's exactly the impression I want you to have. I really do feel like I'm different from other guys. I hate how so many guys treat women like they're expendable ... I also hate when people our age aren't looking for committed relationships. I'm going to be honest with you. I do want a committed relationship. My sole purpose in dating is to find someone to fall in love with and marry. I hope that doesn't scare you."

She said, "That doesn't scare me at all. In fact, I would already have been done with you if I didn't think you'd be a guy that I could be in a relationship with for a long time."

My heart started racing but in the good way. That was the best thing anyone had said to me in months. It was even better to hear that than it was for the nurse to tell me I could leave the hospital. I looked up at the stars briefly and thanked them in my head.

It was starting to get late, and I still had to drive Brittany back to her house, so I asked if she was ready for me to take her home. She nodded her head and told me that she was getting tired anyways.

We got into my car, and when I turned the key in the ignition, my radio turned on automatically. The song "H.O.L.Y." by Florida Georgia Line was on the radio, and it couldn't have been more perfect. I don't think I could have described my feelings any better than that song. Think about it … I was in such a dark place. I felt alone almost every day, and my hope was dwindling. But then, like a miracle, Brittany came into my life, and it was like all the darkness turned to light. The sadness was running away. One date with Brittany, and I didn't feel defeated anymore. I felt like I had finally found the road to recovery.

I didn't want to tell her that yet because I didn't want to put too much pressure on her so fast, but that is how I was feeling. The ride to drop Brittany off at home was quiet because she fell asleep holding my arm in the passenger seat. Normally, if someone falls asleep on the first date, it might be cause for concern, but it was pretty adorable. I perceived it as a sign that she was comfortable around me.

After the forty-minute drive, we arrived in her driveway. She opened her eyes a little disoriented and apologized for falling asleep. I laughed and said, "It's no big deal; you looked too peaceful to wake up." I got out of the car and walked her up to the door of her house to wish her goodnight.

"I know you're tired, but I just want you to know that I had a wonderful time with you tonight. If you would like, I would love to go on another date soon?"

She smiled at my question and replied, "Of course. I had a good time tonight."

Hearing her say she wanted to go on another date with me was such a great feeling! I gave her a hug and asked, "There is a community picnic in a city that's close to where I live next weekend if you would like to go with me?"

"Sure! Sounds like fun!" she said as she walked into her house.

I drove home with an enormous smile on my face. I knew that it felt way too early to feel the way that I did, but you know how they say that you know when you've met "the one?" I felt that way with Brittany on our first date. It was magical; something I had never felt before. Being with her made me feel like I was in the correct spot.

The week went by like normal. Brittany and I talked every chance we got between work and her summer classes. I drove to pick her up Thursday evening for the community picnic. It was only our second date, but I asked if she would like to meet my family.

I told her that my sister and mom had been begging me all week to meet her because they could see how happy she made me, and she told me that she would love to meet them.

With that in mind, I stopped by my house on the way to the picnic, so my mom and sister could meet Brittany. We walked into the house, and my sister greeted Brittany emphatically by saying, "Oh my gosh, you're so pretty!" Brittany smiled and said, "Thanks! You are, too!"

I introduced Brittany to my mom who told Brittany how I always smiled whenever I talked about her. That probably would have embarrassed most people, but I just nodded in confirmation knowing it was the truth.

My Grandpa Alvin also happened to be at our house, so I was able to introduce Brittany to him. We all talked for a few minutes before I told them that Brittany and I were about to leave to go to the picnic.

As I was walking out the door, my grandpa put his hand on my shoulder. I paused as he looked at me, and I noticed that he had a tear forming in his left eye. He was fighting the tear from falling, and with a whimpering lip, he told me, "You always want to be with your best friend."

It may seem cryptic to most people, but I knew exactly what he meant. I smiled and gave him a hug as I walked out the door. My grandpa's phrase played over and over in my head throughout the rest of the evening. My grandma was obviously his best friend. I believe that he saw a connection between Brittany and I that was similar to what he had with my grandma.

Brittany and I had fun at the community picnic. We played carnival games, ate fair food, and listened to the live music playing. After a few hours of being at the picnic, it was time for me to drive Brittany back home.

My grandpa's words played on repeat in my mind the entire drive. "You always want to be with your best friend."

I may have only been talking to Brittany for about two weeks, but I felt like I had known her my whole life. She was already my best friend. I wanted to always be with her. Almost on queue, "H.O.L.Y." came on the radio once we were about five minutes from Brittany's house.

"I have to tell you something," I said to her as she was getting out of the car. "Before we left for the picnic, my grandpa put his hand on my shoulder and told me something that has been on my mind the entire evening. He told me that 'you always want to be with your best friend.' It sounds cryptic, but I know what he meant by it.

"My grandma was his best friend. They were together for forty-one years before she passed away a few months ago. I know we have only been talking and going on dates for a couple weeks, but I feel that way about you already. I already feel like you're my best friend, and I want what my grandpa had with my grandma. You make me so happy. I feel like I can truly be myself around you. Brittany, will you officially be my girlfriend?"

She smiled really big and nodded her head.

"I would be honored."

I ran over to her with my arms spread wide, and she said, "Now that you're my boyfriend, I better be getting more than a hug."

I put my hand lightly in her hair and pulled her closer for our first kiss. The butterflies were swirling around in my stomach, but I wished her goodnight with the faint sound of "H.O.L.Y." playing in the background.

There is a line in the song where the singer says he no longer needs the stars because the person he is singing to shines for him. Wow! That specific line holds a lot of meaning to this story, doesn't it? Brittany was already every star in my personal night sky. She was the matter that filled the voids of space. She was the light at the end of my dark tunnel. She was the reason for me to look up to the sky and be thankful. She was every reason to appreciate being alive.

I wished Brittany good night and got in my car to drive home. I had another one of my patented conversations with myself on the road. However, this one was overwhelmingly positive and reflecting.

I had come full circle. I went from someone who had his heart broken, mourned the loss of his grandma, was in incredible pain, fatally ill, and extremely depressed to someone who was happy and hopeful within a matter of a couple months.

A relationship might not be a resolution for everyone's problems, but Brittany entering my life was life-changing for me. She showed me that there are genuinely good people in the world. She showed me that there is always a reason to have hope. She may not have said anything about it, but she gave me hope. She gave me the hope of a better future, and that is the most amazing feeling a person can have.

Everyone likes an underdog story where someone faces insurmountable odds and overcomes them. Everyone likes to root for a person that is looking for hope but can't seem to find it because life won't cut them a break.

Most people think that they can't be the one that overcomes the odds, but I will tell you that you can be the underdog. You can overcome anything that you put your mind to. You don't have to wait for good things to happen to you. You'll be surprised at how much potential you have and the power that lies within you when you just believe in yourself.

For all I know, I may have been depressed and lonely for years, but I took the chance and started talking to Brittany, which lead to almost instant happiness. I would have never accomplished that if I didn't believe that I was capable of overcoming the odds. The combination of believing in myself, having hope, and love from family and friends as well as from Brittany is how I defeated depression."

I couldn't help but smile the entire drive home. I felt like I had finally won. I had been losing for months at every game I played, but I finally won. It was the most gratifying feeling I have ever had.

EPILOGUE

That night marked the end of my summer. I learned so much about life in 2016. I learned to appreciate every moment you have on this Earth. Appreciate the good days and the bad. Appreciate the people that love you. Appreciate the people that do you wrong. Appreciate the sun, and appreciate the rain. You have to learn to love the negative aspects of life because they will teach you how to truly appreciate the good aspects of life. Without "bad," there can be no "good."

Appreciate every breath you are blessed with. There will be a moment in all our lives when we take our last breath, so cherish each one you get. The amount of breaths you have during your life is much like the amount of time you have during your life - it is forever-decreasing. You will never be able to gain additional time or breaths. You must make the most out of that which you have been given.

If I didn't come to accept and appreciate the dark cloud that 2016 brought over my head, I would have never been able to appreciate the "clear weather" that I was blessed with after. Although I spent the majority of that year depressed, I wouldn't trade a moment of it for anything. I needed the lessons that I was taught. Pain is the greatest teacher. I hardly get upset about anything anymore because I understand now that things can always be worse.

Despite my happy ending with Brittany, 2016 did bring another tragic event for my family. On my mom's birthday, November 21, my Grandma Pam passed away as well. I awoke to my mom's blood-curdling scream; it was the same one that she released when my Grandma Cheryl had passed. We had found out that my grandma had passed away in a freak accident. I'll spare the details, but it hurt not being able to say "goodbye."

It was tough losing both of my grandmothers in one year. I had spent my whole life up to that point with them both being around for every major event, and the realization that I wouldn't be able to share major moments with them anymore was a difficult idea to process.

Brittany and I both went on to graduate from Wright State in April of 2018. We were both first-generation college graduates, and it was amazing being able to share that moment with such an amazing person. Our parents teamed up and threw us a combined graduation party, so all our family and friends could celebrate our achievement with us.

On July 10 (a few months after graduation), Brittany and I moved away from our parents' homes and into an apartment together. I proposed to Brittany on top of the tower at Cox Arboretum on July 21, and she accepted my proposal while crying, of course.

Brittany and I are now married. Our wedding was on August 10, 2019, which was three years and six days after I asked her to be my girlfriend. I couldn't have picked a better life partner.

Knowing that a lot of good things happened to me after 2016 makes me wish that both of my grandmothers could have been there to witness all of the major events. It would have been nice to see them on the day that Brittany and I graduated college. It would have also been nice to see them at our wedding, but I know they were watching … just from a different angle than everyone else.

The moral of my story is to always try to look at the bright side. Life will bring hard times at some point. You just have to understand that there is meaning and importance to every aspect of it. Appreciate every moment you have on this Earth. Appreciate the beauty that life provides. Appreciate the people that love you and know that even if you feel alone, you're not really alone. There are people that love you and want the best for you. It can be hard to see sometimes when the darkness veils your eyes.

Find it within yourself to find the light to guide your vision. Often, we are unable to see things that are right in front of us because we choose not to see them. Choose to see the good, and choose to appreciate the bad as both are equally important in order to overcome the obstacles that life places before you.

Experiencing traumatic things makes seeing the beauty in life much easier. I appreciate life much more after 2016 than I ever did prior to that year. It's amazing the lessons that life teaches you. It will often not be in the manner that you would prefer it to be taught, but life has a way of humbling us through pain.

Learn to appreciate that pain. *Every scar has a story.* The important thing to note about scars is that they heal. Scars are a symbol of repaired damage. Let your scars tell your story, and realize that if you have scars (either physical, mental, or emotional), they are a symbol that you survived whatever obstacle Life put in your path.

You're stronger than you give yourself credit for. You will never know your limits until you're put to the test. Don't be afraid of a challenge. Don't back down when things get tough. Take a stand. I know it sounds cliché, but there is a reason why "underdog" stories are so popular. Be the underdog. People will root for you to succeed, and nothing feels sweeter than winning in a scenario that you were supposed to lose. One last piece of advice:

NEVER GIVE UP. EVER.

ACKNOWLEDGEMENTS

As a rookie author, I have so many people to thank for encouraging me, supporting me, and guiding me through the process of writing this book. Several times as my story unfolded on the previous pages, I had the opportunity to express my love and appreciation for those close to me. Just in case something was missed …

Brittany: Thank you for loving me and supporting me unconditionally throughout the entire process of this book. Your kind heart and care are always appreciated, and I truly couldn't have written my story without you in it. Thank you for being the hero and appreciating what I have to offer. I love you more than words can describe.

Mom: Thank you for always being there any time I call randomly during the day and being there literally any time that I need you. You're always the person I go to if I need something done because you've always found a way to help. I definitely acquired my philosophical mentality from you. No matter how old I get, I'll always be your "Little Man."

Dad: You taught me how to be a fighter and to never accept defeat. At the same time, you always taught me to never stoop down to someone's level that had done me wrong because that will only hurt me on the inside. I have lost count of how many lessons I've learned from you over the years; I just know that I love and appreciate every one of them.

Celeste: Despite being my younger sister, you've always been my bodyguard. You have come such a long way in life, and strangely, I grew a lot from your teen years. That may sound strange, but what I mean is that I learned how to be patient with people because sometimes, it takes people longer to show what they're capable of becoming. I love you, and you'll always be my "kiddo."

Grandpa Alvin and Grandpa Forest: I grouped both of you in together because you both have filled huge roles as my grandpas. You two are sincerely irreplaceable. I love and appreciate both of you so much for being the amazing men and role models that you are. Both of you have such generous and pure hearts that aren't common in today's world, but I will do everything in my power to spread the love and care that you've both bestowed upon me throughout the course of my life. I love you both.

Dexter Poole and Caleb Rose: I have plenty of friends, but I only consider a handful of them to be brothers to me. Both of you are in the "brother" category. With absolutely no malice pointed at any of my other friends, I want to say that you two were there for me when no one else was. You both let me vent to you on numerous occasions while I was going through the events in this book, and I want you to know that I'd be there for anything either of you ever needed. No matter how far our lives may take us, you'll both always be brothers to me. Thank you both.

Grandma Cheryl and Grandma Pam: I know that neither of you will be able to physically see this, but I want you to know that you both played major roles in inspiring me to write this book. Words cannot express how much I miss both of you. I have moments all the time when I'll just randomly miss both of you and want to call you up and tell you about something that happened, but ultimately, I know that you see everything from a better point of view than I could tell it from. I love and miss you both dearly.

Brittany's family: Instead of trying to individually name each of you, I want you all to know that I have appreciated all of you since the moment I met you. You've all welcomed me into the family with open arms since day one, and that kind of acceptance is hard to find. I love all of you, and I'm honored to be a part of such a wonderful family.

Uncle Todd: Todd, you and I have always been close and have shared a connection since I was young. We've witnessed a lot of things go sideways over the years and have always done our best to stick together as a family. That's what family is about, and I just want you to know that I'll always be here if you need me, and I know you'd do the same.

Sandra Combs: Thank you so much for mentoring me through this process and believing in my story enough to want to help me make it as good as it can possibly be. Your guidance, care, and experience has been greatly appreciated, and I look forward to consulting you with my future writing adventures.

Beta Readers, other Family and Friends: Thank you all for being interested in my story and for providing me with feedback before the book went live, support after it went live, and for helping to share my story now with others. Your support and love goes a long way, and I want you all to know that it does not go unnoticed.

ABOUT THE AUTHOR

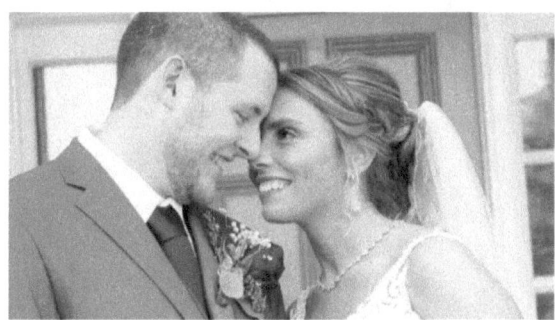

Forest Runnels, and his wife Brittany, graduated from Wright State University in April, 2018 and began their married life together in August, 2019.

Forest is passionate about using his voice to help those struggling with depression. Embedded in the previous pages are words of hope and wisdom from someone who has "been there, done that" when it comes to facing a battle against depression.

Finding an outlet for his thoughts and creativity has been part of Forest's journey. He manages a YouTube Channel titled "Run Forest Runnels" where he shares humor, music, and life advice.

In addition to starting his career, family, and journey as an author, Forest would love to find additional ways to spread his message of hope to those who struggle.

www.ingramcontent.com/pod-product-compliance
Lightning Source LLC
Chambersburg PA
CBHW030706220526
45463CB00005B/1923